THE TOBACCO ATLAS

THIRD EDITION

D1244984

IN MEMORY OF

JUDITH D. WILKENFELD (1943–2007) AND RONALD M. DAVIS (1956–2008)

FOR THEIR LIFETIME ACHIEVEMENTS IN BATTLING THE TOBACCO PANDEMIC

ALSO PUBLISHED BY THE
AMERICAN CANCER SOCIETY

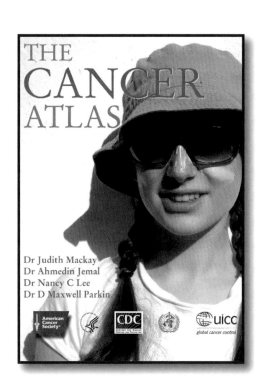

THE TOBACCO ATLAS

THIRD EDITION

DR. OMAR SHAFEY

DR. MICHAEL ERIKSEN

DR. HANA ROSS

DR. JUDITH MACKAY

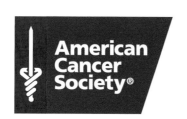
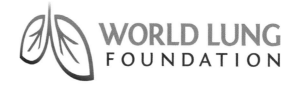

PUBLISHED BY THE AMERICAN CANCER SOCIETY

250 Williams Street
Atlanta, Georgia 30303 USA
www.cancer.org

6 5 4 3 2 09 10 11 12 13

ISBN-10: 1-60443-013-3
ISBN-13: 978-1-60443-013-4
Product Code: 967401

Library of Congress Cataloging-in-Publication Data

The tobacco atlas / authors, Omar Shafey ... [et al.]. —3rd ed.
  p. cm.
Includes bibliographical references and index.
ISBN-13: 978-1-60443-013-4 (pbk. : alk. paper)
ISBN-10: 1-60443-013-3 (pbk. : alk. paper)
1. Tobacco use—Maps. 2. Tobacco industry—Maps. 3. Tobacco—Health aspects—Maps. 4. Medical geography—Maps. I. Shafey, Omar. II. World Health Organization.

G1046.J94T6 2009
362.29'60223—dc22
                            2009000908

Produced for the American Cancer Society by
Bookhouse Group, Inc.
818 Marietta Street, NW, Atlanta, GA 30318, USA
www.bookhouse.net

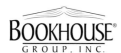

Editorial Director: Rob Levin
Publisher: Barry Levin
Managing Editor and Project Director: Sarah Edwards Fedota
Design Direction, Cartography, and Graphics: Tony De Feria
Design Associate: Alejandro Garay
Design Associate and Prepress: Jill Dible
Copyediting and Indexing: Bob Land
Data Editing: Renee Peyton and Rebecca Robinson
Translations: Transperfect and Antler Translation Services Inc.
International Editions Design: Transperfect

Printed in Canada

CONTENTS

CONTENTS

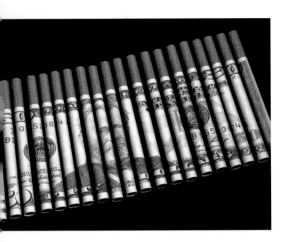

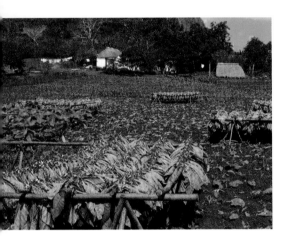

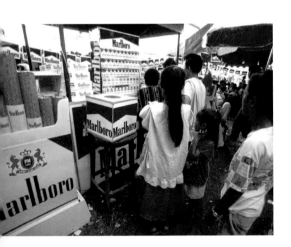

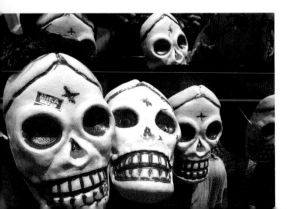

CONTENTS

FOREWORD

The **LIVESTRONG** movement commends the American Cancer Society and World Lung Foundation for taking action in the fight for global tobacco control with their publication of *The Tobacco Atlas*, 3rd edition.

Tobacco accounts for one out of every 10 deaths worldwide and will claim 5.5 million lives this year alone. By 2030, that number is estimated to grow to more than 8 million deaths from tobacco. And that's a tragedy, because those deaths are preventable.

Our friend Mayor Michael R. Bloomberg has shown us with his successful policies in New York City that tobacco control not only saves lives but is also good for business. In cities and states all over America, people are pushing secondhand smoke out of public places. Over half the states and the District of Columbia are enacting comprehensive smoke-free workplace measures. But we can't stop there.

A global challenge like tobacco control requires a global approach. By effectively implementing the World Health Organization Framework Convention on Tobacco Control and MPOWER strategies, we could see a much-needed turning point in reducing tobacco use and its devastating consequences around the world.

It is time to put the interests of public health ahead of the interests of the tobacco companies. Countless lives, our Earth, and the global economy will all be healthier because of it.

Lance Armstrong, Chairman and Founder, Lance Armstrong Foundation

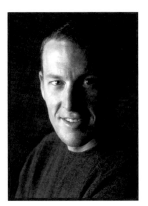

Lance Armstrong

Congratulations to the American Cancer Society and the World Lung Foundation for producing *The Tobacco Atlas*, 3rd edition, a powerful display of the toll tobacco takes globally.

As Mayor of New York City, I know firsthand that this epidemic can be reversed. By raising tobacco taxes, running hard-hitting public information campaigns, creating comprehensive smoke-free public places, and helping people to quit, we have lowered the smoking rate from 21.5 percent to 15.8 percent in only six years. New York City thus has 350,000 fewer smokers, a record decline that could prevent more than 115,000 premature deaths in future years.

Our city's results, along with the large number of deaths in low- and middle-income countries, inspired me to make this fight global. Through Bloomberg Philanthropies, joined by the Bill & Melinda Gates Foundation, we have committed $500 million to a worldwide effort to stop this epidemic. We are focusing on countries such as China and India, where more than one-third of the world's smokers live.

We hope our commitments will help governments confront the tobacco epidemic by implementing strategies including those that worked in New York. Implementation of WHO's MPOWER package is the key to stopping the tobacco epidemic.

Millions of lives can be saved if we act now.

Michael Bloomberg, Mayor, City of New York

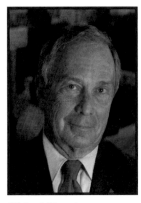

Michael Bloomberg

FOREWORD

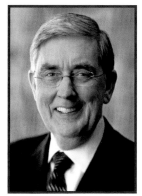
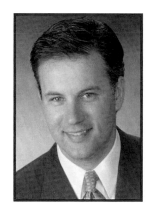

John Seffrin   Peter Baldini

Tobacco is the only consumer product that harms every person exposed to it and kills half of its regular users. Approximately 650 million smokers alive today—10 percent of the current world population—will eventually succumb to tobacco-related disease. An increasing proportion of those deaths will occur in low- and middle-income countries, which will be faced with the severe consequences of the epidemic's financial, social, and political effects.

Yet this extraordinary level of suffering and death is not inevitable. With comprehensive and concerted action, we can reduce or eliminate many of the dangers associated with tobacco, and in so doing, we can save hundreds of millions of lives.

Thanks to the rigorous educational, scientific, and advocacy-based efforts of dedicated tobacco control advocates worldwide, many nations are taking steps to limit the dangerous effects of tobacco, including supporting the world's first global public health treaty—the Framework Convention on Tobacco Control (FCTC). In fact, at least 160 countries have already ratified the treaty and are beginning to implement and enforce its provisions. The World Health Organization's MPOWER strategy, launched in 2008, also provides a proven roadmap for what policymakers, advocates, and public health practitioners can do to combat this global menace.

The six MPOWER strategies are:
- Monitor tobacco use and prevention policies
- Protect people from tobacco smoke
- Offer help to quit tobacco use
- Warn about the dangers of tobacco
- Enforce bans on tobacco advertising, promotion, and sponsorship
- Raise taxes on tobacco

In the comprehensive MPOWER report distributed to governments and leaders throughout the world, WHO established that only 5 percent of the world's population live in countries that fully protect their population with any one of the key measures that reduce smoking rates. The report also found that tobacco taxes, the single most effective strategy, could be significantly increased in nearly all countries, providing a source of sustainable funding to implement and enforce the recommended approach, the package of six MPOWER policies.

With the publication of *The Tobacco Atlas*, 3rd edition, we take another important step toward better informing and empowering the tobacco control community. This timely, evidence-based publication offers compelling data to help governments and tobacco control advocates inform the public about how tobacco is marketed, sold, and consumed in their countries. Now completely revised with up-to-date information and a new online component, *The Tobacco Atlas* exemplifies our progress against tobacco and paves the way for greater strides in the future. Most importantly, this publication helps enable a broad network of policymakers, advocates, and public health practitioners to continue their lifesaving efforts.

Tobacco is a serious foe. But armed with comprehensive information like that found in *The Tobacco Atlas*, we are better prepared to repel the industry's relentless assault and move ever closer to a day when we can finally declare victory over tobacco.

John Seffrin, CEO, American Cancer Society
Peter Baldini, CEO, World Lung Foundation

REVIEWS

Reviews of previous editions of *The Tobacco Atlas*

"*The Tobacco Atlas* is the best thing of its kind I've ever seen."

—C. Everett Koop, Former U.S. Surgeon General

"Informative, so easy to read, beautiful to look at."

—Dr. Annie J. Sasco

"I profited from reading the 2006 second edition of *The Tobacco Atlas.*"

—Dr. R. F. Gillum, Faith-Based and Community Organizations, Centers for Disease Control and Prevention

"It's really helpful and an informative guide for tobacco control advocates."

—Syed Mahbubul Alam Tahin

"Excellent."

—Professor Gérard Dubois

"A comprehensive, attractively produced profile of all major aspects of the tobacco epidemic and what has been done so far to try to reduce it."

—David Simpson

"A manual of immense value for all people involved in smoking control."

—Dr. Kjell Bjartveit

"A beautiful and informative book."

—Professor Tai Hing Lam, Department of Community Medicine, University of Hong Kong

"We are making an addictive product that causes death and diseases among smokers. But we know, and *The Tobacco Atlas* points this out, that smoking will continue. People will continue to smoke, and something needs to be done about it."

—Chris Nelson, Manager, Regulatory Affairs, Philip Morris Asia

PREFACE

The Tobacco Atlas is intended for readers interested in the effect tobacco has on health, politics, economics, big business, corporate behavior, globalization, smuggling, tax, religion, allocation of resources, poverty, gender issues, human rights, children, human development, and the future.

This third edition of *The Tobacco Atlas* maps the history, documents the current situation, and predicts the future of the tobacco epidemic. The chapters illustrate that tobacco is not simply a matter of personal choice, but also involves a political and economic panoply of global social and demographic change, government policy, and corporate strategies, including tobacco industry activities such as smuggling, deceptive marketing, and evasion of corporate responsibility. This Atlas reflects the importance of multilateral approaches to reduce the epidemic, requiring action by the World Health Organization, other UN agencies, governmental and non-governmental organizations (NGOs), the private sector, and concerned individuals—in fact, the whole of civil society.

Since the previous edition of *The Tobacco Atlas* was published in 2006, there have been several significant developments in global tobacco control. To date, 162 countries have ratified the WHO Framework Convention on Tobacco Control, the first application of international law to further public health. In 2008, the World Health Organization issued the MPOWER report, a comprehensive analysis of global tobacco use and control efforts. The MPOWER report provides an unprecedented level of detail and a roadmap for effective solutions. The recent contributions of major international donors, such as the Bloomberg Philanthropies and the Bill & Melinda Gates Foundation, have improved the global tobacco control environment by significantly increasing levels of funding for tobacco control efforts in low-and middle-resource countries.

As the costs of tobacco have been more carefully studied in different national economies, policy makers and the public are realizing that tobacco control benefits the health and wealth of nations and individuals. More countries have passed legislation to increase tobacco taxes, ban tobacco promotion, require health warnings, and create smoke-free areas in public places. In many countries, tobacco industry documents are being analyzed to expose the harmful activities of the tobacco industry and hold it responsible for damages. The most effective national tobacco control plans integrate comprehensive tobacco control activities into existing health and education programs.

Despite progress in policy development and public awareness, the world's total number of smokers and the number of tobacco-related deaths continues to grow. This unfortunate trend, due largely to global population increases, is likely to continue for the foreseeable future. Tragically, the tobacco burden is falling increasingly on low- and middle-resource countries, and the concern that more women are smoking cannot be underestimated.

The publication of this third edition of the atlas marks a critical juncture in the unfolding pandemic. With an eye on the past century and the remainder of this century ahead, we can choose to stand by idly while the tobacco industry causes another one billion deaths in the twenty-first century, or we can embrace the spirit of the Framework Convention on Tobacco Control by implementing robust and effective measures to protect people's health and the wealth of nations. Millions of lives, trillions of dollars, and the world's prospects for an equitable future hang in the balance.

Omar Shafey, Scientific Integrity Consulting LLC, Atlanta, USA
Michael Eriksen, Georgia State University, Atlanta, USA
Hana Ross, American Cancer Society, Atlanta, USA
Judith Mackay, World Lung Foundation, Hong Kong, SAR China

ACKNOWLEDGMENTS

Sincere thanks to the American Cancer Society and the World Lung Foundation for their generous financial support of the third edition of *The Tobacco Atlas*. This version of the atlas has been revised from a previous version released earlier in 2009. An online version of this atlas is available at www.TobaccoAtlas.org. Many people have helped in the preparation of this atlas. First, we especially would like to thank our principal researchers: Denyse N. C. Nanan, International Affairs Department, American Cancer Society; Samina Shariff, Epidemiology and Surveillance Research, American Cancer Society; Lindsay J. Feldman, Dena Elimam, Katie Elizabeth Brown, and Su Su, International Affairs Department, American Cancer Society; Allison Edwards and Megan Reynolds, Institute of Public Health, Georgia State University; and Ellie Rampton, World Lung Foundation.

We would like to thank our peers who reviewed the second edition and made suggestions for the third edition of *The Tobacco Atlas*: Cathy Backinger, National Cancer Institute; Kelley Lee, London School of Hygiene and Tropical Medicine; Prakash C. Gupta, Healis - Sekhsaria Institute for Public Health; Martin Raw, University of Nottingham; Lawrence O. Gostin, Georgetown University; Eric LeGresley, Anne-Marie Perucic, Tobacco Free Initiative, WHO; Majid Ezzati, Harvard University; Ana Navas-Acien, Johns Hopkins Bloomberg School of Public Health; Rosemary Kennedy, Research for International Tobacco Control, International Development Research Center, Canada; Nancy Lee, Division of Cancer Prevention and Control, Centers for Disease Control and Prevention; Sverre Berg Lutnæs, Norwegian Cancer Society; Derek Yach, PepsiCo; Heidi Tjugum, Norwegian Cancer Society; Emmanuel Guindon, McMaster University; Phan Thi Hai, VINACOSH Standing Office, Ministry of Health, Vietnam; Hatai Chitanondh, the National Health Foundation, Thailand; and Tom Frieden, Kelly Henning, Jennifer Ellis, and Neena Prasad, Bloomberg Initiative to Reduce Tobacco Use.

Additional acknowledgment goes to the World Health Organization for providing data from the MPOWER report (2008) used in several spreads.

We acknowledge the contribution of the first and second editions of the atlas to this third edition, especially the World Health Organization, publishers of the first edition of *The Tobacco Atlas*; Myriad Editions, the packager for the first and second editions; and other contributors who helped shape the previous atlas editions.

We would like to thank the following staff from the American Cancer Society for researching, revising, and helping re-release this third edition: Greg Guthrie, Corporate Communications; Catherine Jo, International Affairs Department; Rennie Sloan, Corporate Communications; Cassandra Welch, International Affairs Department. We would also like to thank the following staff from World Lung Foundation for their guidance in design, editing, artwork, distribution, and promotion of this edition: Jorge Alday, Yvette Chang, Stephen Hamill, Alexey Kotov, Mego Lien, Sandra Mullin.

We would like to thank the staff at Bookhouse Group, Inc., including Rob Levin, Renee Peyton, Jill Dible, Bob Land, Tony De Feria, the translation teams, international design firm, and other team members who worked on this edition of the atlas. Special recognition goes to Sarah Fedota, Bookhouse Group managing editor, who received a diagnosis of lung cancer while working on the atlas. A lifelong nonsmoker exposed to secondhand smoke, Sarah's poignant struggle, strength, and dignity as a cancer survivor serve as an inspiration to all.

For their advice on particular maps and subjects, we would like to thank the following individuals:

1 Types of Tobacco Use

Samira Asma, Centers for Disease Control and Prevention, USA

Prakash Gupta, Healis - Sekhsaria Institute of Public Health, Mumbai, India

2 Male Smoking

Michael Thun, Department of Epidemiology and Surveillance Research, American Cancer Society

Yumiko Mochizuki-Kobayashi, Japan Ministry of Health and Welfare

3 Female Smoking

Michael Thun, Department of Epidemiology and Surveillance Research, American Cancer Society

Yumiko Mochizuki-Kobayashi, Japan Ministry of Health and Welfare

5 Boys' Tobacco Use and 6 Girls' Tobacco Use

Wick Warren and Veronica Lea, Office on Smoking and Health, Centers for Disease Control and Prevention, USA

PHOTO CREDITS

The publishers are grateful to the following organizations and photographers for permission to reproduce their photographs:

Part One: Prevalence and Health
- Death clock: AP Images/Laurent Gillieron

Chapter 1: Types of Tobacco Use
- Pair of hands holding bidis: World Lung Foundation
- Three kreteks: Tony De Feria
- Sticks: Tony De Feria

Chapter 2: Male Smoking
- Little boy standing next to sitting man who is smoking: World Lung Foundation/ Gary Hampton

Chapter 3: Female Smoking
- Balloon seller: World Lung Foundation/ Sudipto Das

Chapter 8: Health Risks
- Anatomy figure: Tony De Feria

Part Four: Promotion
- People in front of Marlboro stand: World Health Organization/Jim Holmes

Chapter 17: Marketing
- Lucky Strike: World Lung Foundation/ Damien Schumann

Part Five: Taking Action
- Death masks: World Lung Foundation/ Sudipto Das

Chapter 21: Capacity Building
- Bill Gates: Associated Press/Bebeto Matthews

Chapter 25: Product Labeling
- Plain packaging: The Cancer Council of Western Australia

Chapter 26: Public Health Campaigns
- Non-smoking section: NYC Department of Health and Mental Hygiene
- Publimentro restaurant: Instituto Nacional de Salud Publica
- OOH sponge: Forum of Young Ukrainian Leaders
- Not smokefree: National Tobacco Control Program, Government of India

Part Six: World Tables
- Man smokes while reading to daughter: AP Images/Greg Baker

ABOUT THE AUTHORS

Omar Shafey

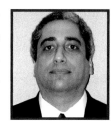

Dr. Omar Shafey, a medical anthropologist and epidemiologist, is managing partner at Scientific Integrity Consulting, LLC and adjunct professor of Global Health at Emory University's Rollins School of Public Health in Atlanta, Georgia, USA. He edited the Tobacco Control Country Profiles 2003, coauthored the second edition of *The Tobacco Atlas*, and has published research on smoking among women in Spain, cigarette smuggling in Brazil, and lung cancer trends among young adults in the USA.

Michael Eriksen

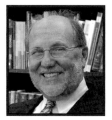

Dr. Michael Eriksen is Professor and founding Director of the Institute of Public Health at Georgia State University. Prior to his current position, Dr. Eriksen served as a Senior Advisor to the World Health Organization in Geneva and was Director of the CDC's Office on Smoking and Health, serving in this capacity from 1992 to 2000. Dr. Eriksen has published extensively on tobacco prevention and control and has served as an expert witness in litigation against the tobacco industry. He is Editor-in-Chief of Health Education Research and has been designated as a Distinguished Cancer Scholar by the Georgia Cancer Coalition. He is a recipient of the WHO Commemorative Medal on Tobacco or Health and a Presidential Citation for Meritorious Service by former President Bill Clinton. He is Past President and Distinguished Fellow of the Society for Public Health Education, and for thirty years he has been a member of the American Public Health Association.

Hana Ross

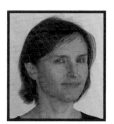

Dr. Hana Ross is an economist and Strategic Director of International Tobacco Control Research at the American Cancer Society. She is also Deputy Director of the International Tobacco Evidence Network (ITEN) and an adjunct professor at both Georgia State University and Emory University in Atlanta, Georgia, USA. She has published extensively on the economics of tobacco control and is a mentor and leader for various research projects in low- and middle-income countries, including projects funded by the World Health Organization, the Rockefeller Foundation, the Open Society Institute, the European Commission, and the Bloomberg Global Initiative. She organizes seminars and teaches economics of tobacco control at regional workshops and serves as a technical advisor to the South East Asia Tobacco Control Alliance.

Judith Mackay

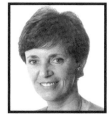

Dr. Judith Longstaff Mackay is a medical doctor based in Hong Kong. She is Senior Advisor to the World Lung Foundation, Senior Policy Advisor to the World Health Organization, and Director of the Asian Consultancy on Tobacco Control. She holds professorships at the Chinese Academy of Preventive Medicine in Beijing and the Department of Community Medicine at the University of Hong Kong. She is a Fellow of the Royal Colleges of Physicians of Edinburgh and of London. After an early career as a hospital physician, she moved to preventive and public health. Dr. Mackay has received many international awards, including the WHO Commemorative Medal, Royal Awards from the United Kingdom's Queen Elizabeth II and Thailand's King Bhumibol Adulyadej, the Fries Prize for Improving Health, the Luther Terry Award for Outstanding Individual Leadership, the International Partnering for World Health Award, the Founding International Achievement Award from the Asia Pacific Association for the Control of Tobacco, and the Lifetime Achievement Award from the International Network of Women Against Tobacco. In 2007, she was selected as one of *Time* magazine's 100 World's Most Influential People. She coauthored the first two editions of *The Tobacco Atlas* and several other health atlases, including *The Penguin Atlas of Human Sexual Behavior*, *The Atlas of Heart Disease and Stroke*, *The State of Health Atlas*, and *The Cancer Atlas*.

GLOSSARY

Addiction – Physiological or psychological dependence on a substance characterized by neurochemical changes, compulsive drug-seeking behavior, dose tolerance, withdrawal symptoms, uncontrolled craving, and self-destructive behavior. Common addictive drugs include alcohol, opiates, and nicotine.

Advertising – Any commercial effort to promote tobacco consumption, including the display of trade-marks, brand names, and manufacturer logos; marketing of tobacco products; sponsorship of sports and other social and cultural activities; and other methods.

BCE – Before the Common Era

Billion – 1,000 million

Bupropion – An antidepressant pharmaceutical used as a smoking cessation aid. A norepinephrine and dopamine reuptake inhibitor as well as a nicotinic antagonist, bupropion was first approved for smoking cessation in 1997.

Cancer – A type of disease in which abnormal cells divide uncontrollably. Cancer cells can invade nearby tissues and spread through the bloodstream and lymphatic system to other parts of the body. Tobacco consumption significantly increases incidence and mortality due to many types of cancer, especially cancers of the lung and oral cavity. Tobacco is also associated with cancers of the pharynx, larynx, esophagus, pancreas, cervix, kidney, bladder, colon, and other organs.

Carcinogen – A substance that causes cancer. Tobacco contains many potent chemical carcinogens, including tobacco-specific nitrosamines (TSNAs), polyaromatic hydrocarbons (PAHs), and volatile organic compounds (VOCs).

Chronic bronchitis – Inflammation of the bronchial mucous membrane characterized by cough, hypersecretion of mucus, and expectoration of sputum over a long period of time, associated with increased vulnerability to bronchial infection. Smoking greatly increases incidence of chronic bronchitis and risk of death due to respiratory disease.

Chronic obstructive pulmonary disease (COPD) – A chronic lung disease, such as asthma or emphysema, in which breathing becomes slowed or forced. Smoking increases risk of death due to COPD and other respiratory diseases. See also "Chronic bronchitis."

Consumption – Total cigarette consumption is the number of cigarettes sold annually in a country, usually in millions of sticks. Total cigarette consumption is calculated by adding a country's cigarette production and imports and subtracting exports. "Per adult"

cigarette consumption is calculated by dividing total cigarette consumption by the total population of those who are 15 years and older. Smuggling may account for inaccuracies in these estimates.

Contraband – Smuggled, counterfeit, or otherwise illicit products. See also "Illicit trade in tobacco products."

Coronary artery disease – Also known as coronary heart disease. The narrowing or blockage of the coronary arteries (blood vessels that carry blood and oxygen to the heart) usually caused by atherosclerosis (a build-up of fatty material [cholesterol] and plaque inside the coronary arteries). Tobacco consumption greatly increases the incidence and mortality due to coronary artery diseases.

Costs – Macroeconomic costs associated with tobacco use.

> **Direct costs:** Health costs related to diseases caused by tobacco; health-care costs, such as hospital services, physician and outpatient services, prescription drugs, nursing home services, home health care, allied health care; changed expenditures due to increased utilization of services.

> **Indirect costs:** Productivity costs caused by tobacco-related illness or premature death; loss of productivity and earnings.

> **Total costs:** The sum of direct and indirect tobacco-attributable costs to society.

Cotinine – Nicotine's major metabolite. Because cotinine has a significantly longer half-life than nicotine, cotinine measurement can be used to estimate tobacco exposure levels. Cotinine is commonly measured in blood serum, urine, and saliva.

Counterfeit tobacco products – Illegally manufactured cigarettes or other products bearing a trademark without the consent of the trademark owner. See also "Illicit trade in tobacco products."

Emphysema – A pathological condition of the lungs marked by an abnormal increase in the size of the air spaces, resulting in labored breathing and an increased susceptibility to infection. It can be caused by irreversible expansion of the alveoli or by the destruction of alveolar walls. Smoking is a major risk factor for emphysema.

Environmental tobacco smoke (ETS) – See Secondhand smoke (SHS).

Excess mortality – The amount by which death rates for a given population group (e.g., smokers) exceeds that of another population group chosen as a reference or standard (e.g., nonsmokers).

Framework Convention on Tobacco Control – The World Health Organization (WHO) Framework Convention on Tobacco Control (WHO FCTC) is the first global treaty negotiated under the auspices of the World Health Organization. WHO FCTC establishes the international public health and legal template for national tobacco control activities.

Global Youth Tobacco Survey (GYTS) – The World Health Organization (WHO) and the Centers for Disease Control and Prevention (CDC) developed the GYTS to track tobacco use among young people across countries using a common methodology and core questionnaire.

GNI – Gross national income.

Harm reduction – A public health philosophy that seeks to mitigate health hazards by replacing high-risk products or activities with lower-risk products or activities. In tobacco control, harm reduction is proposed for smokers who do not want to stop smoking or are unable to do so despite many attempts. Harm reduction seeks to reduce the adverse health effects of smoking by removing harmful constituents or encouraging smokers to switch to alternative modes of tobacco consumption that are considered less harmful than smoking—for example, smokeless tobacco. The approach is controversial because all forms of tobacco consumption are harmful, and medically acceptable smoking cessation approaches do not employ tobacco as a cessation aid.

Health professionals – Dentists, health science practitioners, hospital staff, medical doctors, nurses, pharmacists, ancillary medical staff, and students in these disciplines.

Health warnings – Government-mandated medical statements or graphic images placed on tobacco products, packaging, or advertisements.

Illicit manufacturing – Illegal manufacturing of tobacco products in defiance of tax, licensing, or monopolistic laws that restrict the manufacture of tobacco products. See also "Illicit trade in tobacco products."

Illicit trade in tobacco products – Any practice or conduct prohibited by law, relating to production, shipment, receipt, possession, distribution, sale, or purchase of tobacco products, including any practice or conduct intended to facilitate such activity. See also "Contraband, Counterfeit tobacco products, Illicit manufacturing, and Smuggling."

Ingredient – Every component of the tobacco product that is smoked or chewed, including all genetically modified, blended, and introduced components, additives, flavorings, and other constituents, including paper, ink, adhesives, hardening agents, filters, and other materials used in the manufacturing process and present in the finished product in burned or unburned form.

Marketing – A range of activities aimed at ensuring the continued sales and profitability of a product, including advertising, promotion, public relations, and sales.

Nicotiana tabacum – The tobacco plant. Its leaves contain high levels of the addictive chemical nicotine and many cancer-causing chemicals, especially polyaromatic hydrocarbons (PAHs). The leaves may be smoked (in cigarettes, cigars, and pipes), applied to the gums (as dipping and chewing tobacco), or inhaled (as snuff). Tobacco use and exposure to secondhand tobacco smoke causes many types of cancer, as well as heart, respiratory, and other diseases.

Nicotine – An addictive, poisonous alkaloid chemical found in tobacco. It is also a stimulant that increases heart rate and oxygen use by cardiac muscle. Nicotine is also used as an insecticide. The lethal dose for a human adult is about 50mg.

Nicotine replacement therapy (NRT) – A type of smoking cessation treatment that provides low doses of nicotine to ease cravings experienced by addicted smokers. NRTs include devices such as transdermal patches, nicotine gum, nicotine nasal sprays, and inhalers.

Passive smoking – Inhaling cigarette, cigar, or pipe smoke produced by another individual. See also "Secondhand smoke (SHS)."

Polyaromatic hydrocarbon (PAH) – A type of organic compound composed of several benzene rings. PAHs, many of which are carcinogenic, are produced during charbroiling of meat, incomplete combustion of fossil fuels, and the burning of tobacco. Tobacco smoke is the most common source of human exposure.

Prevalence – Smoking prevalence is the percentage of smokers in the total population. Adult smoking prevalence is usually defined as the percentage of smokers among those aged 15 years and older.

Promotion – Special offers, gifts, price discounts, coupons, company Web sites, specialty item distribution, telephone solicitation, and other methods to facilitate the sale or placement of cigarettes. Also includes allowances paid to cigarette retailers, wholesalers, full-time company employees, and all other persons involved in cigarette distribution.

Retailer – A person engaged in a business that includes the sale of tobacco products to consumers.

Risk – The likelihood of incurring a particular event or circumstance (e.g., risk of disease measures the chance of an individual contracting a disease).

Secondhand smoke (SHS) – Smoke inhaled by an individual not actively engaged in smoking. SHS is composed of mainstream smoke (exhaled by smokers) and sidestream smoke (from the tip of the cigarette, cigar, or pipe). Secondhand smoke contains the same harmful chemicals that smokers inhale. Also known as environmental tobacco smoke (ETS) or passive smoking.

Smoke-free area – Area where smoking or holding a lighted cigarette, cigar, or pipe is prohibited.

Smokeless tobacco – Snuff, chewing tobacco, and other forms of tobacco used orally; not a safe alternative to smoking. Smokeless tobacco is as addictive as smoking, and it causes cancer of the gum, cheek, lip, mouth, tongue, and throat.

Smoker – Someone who smokes any tobacco product either daily or occasionally.

Smuggling – The illegal importation of products. See also "Illicit trade in tobacco products."

> **Large-scale organized smuggling of tobacco products:** illegal transportation, distribution, and sale of large consignments of cigarettes and other tobacco products.

> **Small-scale smuggling or "bootlegging":** individual or small group purchases of tobacco products in low-price jurisdictions in amounts that exceed the limits set by customs regulations, for resale in high-price jurisdictions.

Stroke – An abnormal condition in which a blood vessel in the brain bursts or is clogged by a blood clot leading to the death of brain cells. Strokes usually result in temporary or permanent neurological deficits and/or death. Smoking significantly increases the risk of stroke.

Tar – The raw anhydrous nicotine-free condensate of smoke.

Tar and nicotine yield – The amount of tar and nicotine in one cigarette, as determined by a machine designed to measure the chemical content of cigarette smoke. Machine yields of cigarette tar and nicotine levels may not reflect the actual level of exposure experienced by smokers. See also "Tobacco smoke condensate."

Tobacco attributable mortality – The number of deaths attributable to tobacco use within a specific population.

Tobacco control organization – A nonprofit organization with a goal of reducing tobacco consumption or protecting nonsmokers from the effects of secondhand smoke.

Tobacco industry documents – Previously secret, internal industry records that are now available in the public domain as a result of court rulings.

Tobacco product – Any product manufactured wholly or partly from tobacco that is ingested by smoking, inhalation, chewing, sniffing, or sucking.

Tobacco production – The volume of actual tobacco leaves harvested from the field, excluding harvesting and threshing losses and any part of the unharvested tobacco crop.

Tobacco smoke condensate (TSC) – Sticky particles comprising thousands of chemicals created by burning tobacco.

Tobacco-specific nitrosamine (TSN or TSNA) – A group of seven toxic chemicals found only in tobacco products. N'-nitrosonornicotine (NNN), (4-methylnitrosamino)-1-(3-pyridyl)-1-butanone (NNK), and N-oxide, 4-(methylnitrosamino)-1-(3-pyridyl N-oxide)-1-butanol (NNAL; a metabolic product of NNK) are the most carcinogenic.

Tobacco taxes – The sum of all types of taxes levied on tobacco products. There are two basic methods of tobacco taxation:

> **Nominal or specific taxes:** Based on a set amount of tax per unit (e.g., cigarette) or gram of tobacco. These taxes are often differentiated according to the type of tobacco product (e.g., filtered vs. nonfiltered cigarettes, pipe tobacco vs. cigars).

> **Ad valorem taxes:** Assessed as a percentage markup on some determined value (tax base), usually the retail selling price of tobacco products or a wholesale price. These taxes include any value-added tax (VAT) where applicable.

Tobacco use – The consumption of tobacco products by burning, chewing, inhalation, or other forms of ingestion.

Varenicline – A pharmaceutical smoking cessation aid that acts as a partial agonist of nicotinic acetylcholine receptors. It became available beginning in 2006.

Volatile organic compound (VOC) – An organic (carbon-containing) compound that evaporates at room temperature. VOCs contribute significantly to indoor air pollution and respiratory disease.

397

PART ONE

PREVALENCE AND HEALTH

"Every number was a family member and a loved one."

— Mary Assunta, head of the Framework Convention Alliance. The Alliance's "death clock" started when countries began negotiating the framework convention on October 25, 1999, and has since tallied more than 39,779,710 dead of tobacco-related diseases.

CHAPTER 1

TYPES OF TOBACCO USE

Cigarettes account for the largest share of manufactured tobacco products in the world—96 percent of total sales. Except for chewing tobacco in India and smoking of kreteks in Indonesia, cigarettes are the most common method of consuming tobacco throughout the world.

The invention of the cigarette-rolling machine in 1881 accelerated the tobacco pandemic by mass-producing pocket-sized packets of cigarettes. Unlike tediously hand-rolled cigarettes and bulky water pipes, manufactured cigarettes offered a convenient and portable method to maintain addiction, even while driving a motor vehicle, working in a factory, or taking a stroll.

In the current era of economic globalization, some forms of tobacco, historically localized to specific regions of the world (such as the hookah and bidi), have spread to every continent. For instance, Indonesian kreteks—clove-flavored, loosely packed tobacco cigarettes—are currently being marketed to youth in many industrialized countries. These regional forms of tobacco sometimes gain footholds in new countries based on their exotic cachet, but they rarely, if ever, displace manufactured cigarettes for a significant market share. Instead, they frequently serve as a gateway to addiction, luring youth and other fad smokers into lifelong dependence on cigarettes.

 THERE IS NO safe way to use tobacco—whether inhaled, sniffed, sucked, or chewed; whether some of the harmful ingredients are reduced; or whether it is mixed with other ingredients.

Smokeless tobacco

Smokeless tobacco is usually consumed orally or nasally, without burning or combustion. There are two main types of smokeless tobacco: snuff and chewing tobacco.

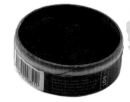

DRY SNUFF

Dry snuff is powdered tobacco that is inhaled through the nose and absorbed through the nasal mucosa or taken orally. Once widespread, particularly in Europe, the use of dry snuff is in decline.

Most Prevalent: *Europe*

MOIST SNUFF

Moist snuff is a small amount of ground tobacco held in the mouth between the cheek and gum. Manufacturers are increasingly prepackaging moist snuff into small paper or cloth packets to make the product more convenient. Other moist snuff products are known as khaini, snus, shammaah, nass, or naswa.

Most Prevalent: *Worldwide*

CHEWING TOBACCO

Oral smokeless tobacco products are placed in the mouth, cheek, or inner lip and sucked (dipped) or chewed. Tobacco pastes or powders are similarly used, placed 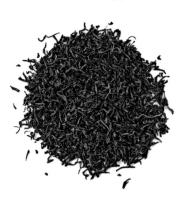 on the gums or teeth. Sometimes referred to as "spit tobacco" because users spit out the built-up tobacco juices and saliva, this mode of tobacco consumption became associated with American baseball players during the twentieth century. The tobacco industry exploited these sports heroes to market their tobacco products to youth. Smokeless tobacco causes cancer in humans and leads to nicotine addiction similar to that produced by cigarette smoking.

There are many varieties of smokeless tobacco, including plug, loose-leaf, chimo, toombak, gutkha, and twist. Pan masala or betel quid consists of tobacco, areca nuts (*Areca catechu*), slaked lime (calcium hydroxide), sweeteners, and flavoring agents wrapped in a betel leaf (*Piper betel*). There are endless varieties of pan masala, including kaddipudi, hogesoppu, gundi, kadapam, zarda, pattiwala, kiwam, and mishri.

Most Prevalent: *India*

Smoking tobacco

Tobacco smoking is the act of burning dried or cured leaves of the tobacco plant and inhaling the smoke.
Combustion releases biochemically active compounds in tobacco, such as nicotine and TSNA, and allows them to be absorbed through the lungs.

ROLL-YOUR-OWN

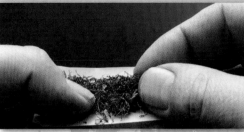

Roll-your-own (RYO) cigarettes are cigarettes hand-filled by the smoker from fine-cut, loose tobacco rolled in a cigarette paper. RYO cigarette smokers are exposed to high concentrations of tobacco particulates, tar, nicotine, and tobacco-specific nitrosamines (TSNAs), and are at increased risk for developing cancers of the mouth, pharynx, larynx, lung, and esophagus.

Most Prevalent: *Europe and New Zealand*

MANUFACTURED CIGARETTES

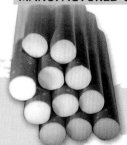

Manufactured cigarettes are the most commonly consumed tobacco products worldwide. They consist of shredded or reconstituted tobacco, processed with hundreds of chemicals and rolled into a paper-wrapped cylinder. Usually tipped with a cellulose acetate filter, they are lit at one end and inhaled through the other.

Most Prevalent: *Worldwide*

CIGARS

Cigars are made of air-cured and fermented tobaccos with a tobacco-leaf wrapper. The long aging and fermentation process produces high concentrations of carcinogenic compounds that are released on combustion. The concentrations of toxins and irritants in cigars are higher than in cigarettes. Cigars come in many shapes and sizes, from cigarette-sized cigarillos to double coronas, cheroots, stumpen, chuttas, and dhumtis. In reverse chutta and dhumti smoking, the ignited end of the cigar is placed inside the mouth.

Most Prevalent: *Worldwide*

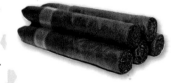

BIDIS

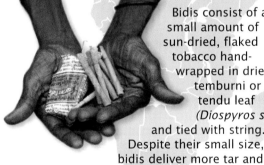

Bidis consist of a small amount of sun-dried, flaked tobacco hand-wrapped in dried temburni or tendu leaf *(Diospyros sp.)* and tied with string. Despite their small size, bidis deliver more tar and carbon monoxide than manufactured cigarettes because users are forced to puff harder to keep bidis lit. Bidis are found throughout South Asia and are the most heavily consumed smoked tobacco products in India.

Most Prevalent: *South Asia*

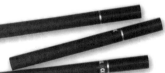

KRETEKS

Kreteks are clove-flavored cigarettes widely smoked in Indonesia. They may contain a wide range of exotic flavorings and eugenol, which has an anesthetic effect, allowing for deeper and more harmful smoke inhalation.

Most Prevalent: *Indonesia*

WATER PIPES

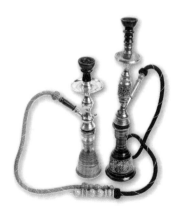

Water pipes, also known as shisha, hookah, narghile, or hubble-bubble, operate by water filtration and indirect heat. Flavored tobacco is burned in a smoking bowl covered with foil and coal. The smoke is cooled by filtration through a basin of water and consumed through a hose and mouthpiece.

Most Prevalent: *North Africa, the Mediterranean region, and parts of Asia.*

PIPES

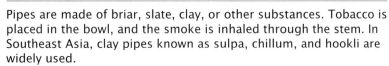

Pipes are made of briar, slate, clay, or other substances. Tobacco is placed in the bowl, and the smoke is inhaled through the stem. In Southeast Asia, clay pipes known as sulpa, chillum, and hookli are widely used.

Most Prevalent: *Worldwide*

STICKS

Sticks are made from sun-cured tobacco and wrapped in cigarette paper—for example, hand-rolled brus.

Most Prevalent: *Papua New Guinea*

CHAPTER 2

MALE SMOKING

"As a man who smoked regularly for 45 years . . . I feel I should inform the future smokers that to smoke means to write off part of your own freedom."
—VÁCLAV HAVEL, PRESIDENT OF THE CZECH REPUBLIC, 2000

Smoking is marketed as a masculine habit, linked to health, happiness, fitness, wealth, power, and virility. In reality, it leads to sickness, premature death, sexual impotence, and infertility.

Almost 1 billion men in the world smoke—about 35 percent of men in high-resource countries, and 50 percent of men in developing countries. Male smoking rates have now peaked, and trends in low- and middle-resource countries indicate slow but sure declines. However, this extremely slow trend is progressing over decades while, in the meantime, tobacco is killing about 5 million men every year. In general, higher-educated men are abandoning tobacco addiction, leaving the smoking habit to poorer, less-educated men.

China deserves special mention because of the enormity of the tobacco problem and the danger it poses. Nearly 60 percent of Chinese men are smokers, and the country consumes more than 37 percent of the world's cigarettes. China's monumental addiction is, according to Philip Morris, "the most important feature on the landscape." Escalating health and economic tolls imposed by tobacco threaten to impede the stable development of this major world power.

"It is more important to concentrate on strong masculine user imagery than to risk diluting this image with low tar."

—R. J. Reynolds internal memorandum, 1980

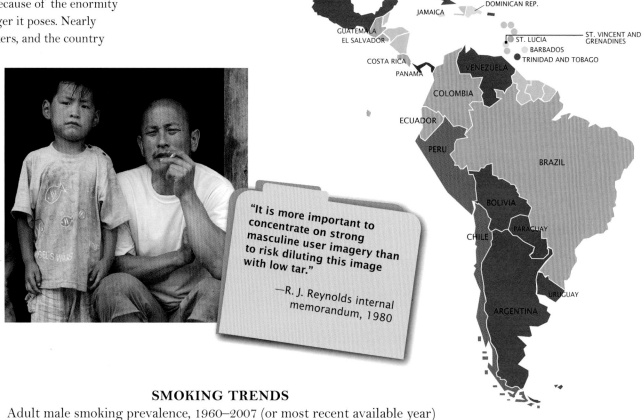

SMOKING TRENDS

Adult male smoking prevalence, 1960–2007 (or most recent available year)

United States

52% '65
44% '70
38% '79
28% '90
26% '00
24% '06
23% '07

United Kingdom

61% '60
55% '70
42% '80
31% '90
29% '00
23% '06

Japan

81% '60
78% '70
70% '80
61% '90
54% '00
40% '06/'07

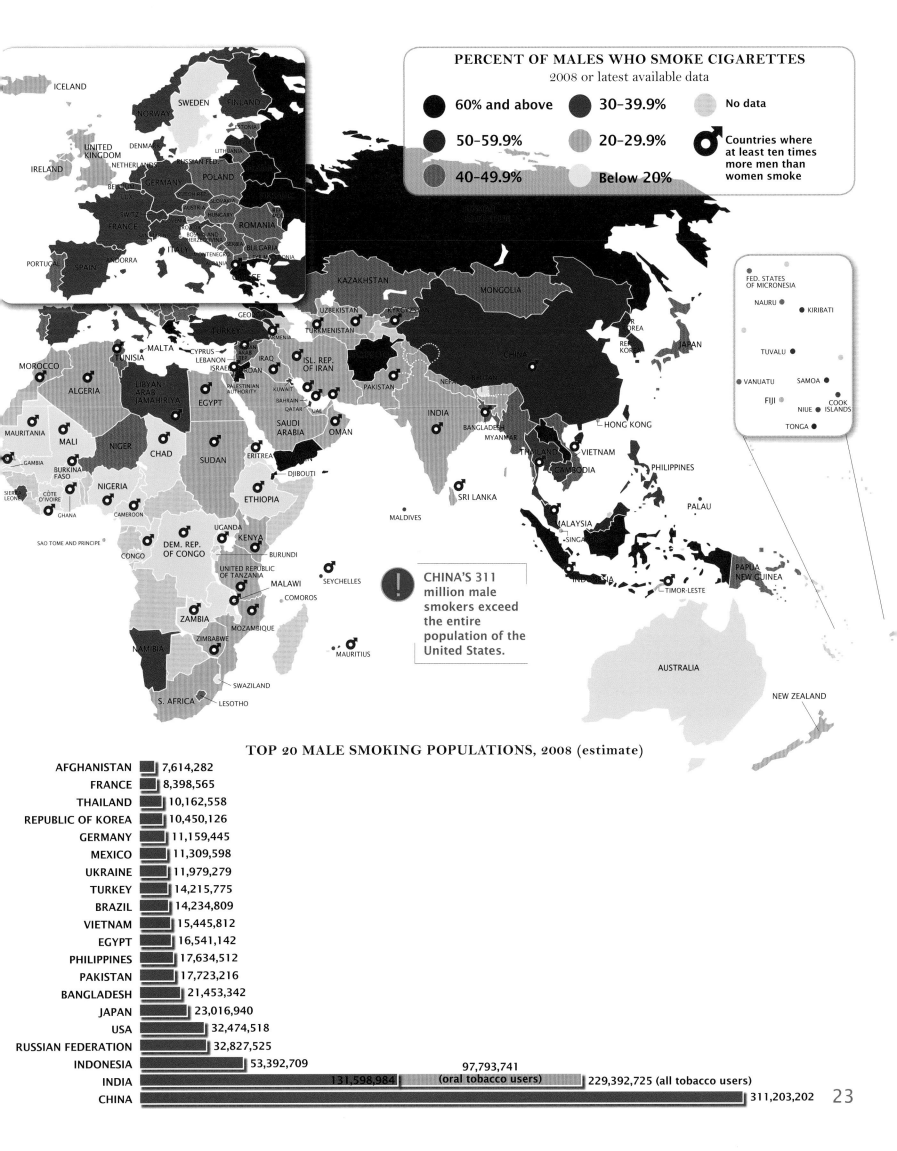

PERCENT OF MALES WHO SMOKE CIGARETTES
2008 or latest available data

- 60% and above
- 50-59.9%
- 40-49.9%
- 30-39.9%
- 20-29.9%
- Below 20%
- No data
- Countries where at least ten times more men than women smoke

CHINA'S 311 million male smokers exceed the entire population of the United States.

TOP 20 MALE SMOKING POPULATIONS, 2008 (estimate)

AFGHANISTAN	7,614,282
FRANCE	8,398,565
THAILAND	10,162,558
REPUBLIC OF KOREA	10,450,126
GERMANY	11,159,445
MEXICO	11,309,598
UKRAINE	11,979,279
TURKEY	14,215,775
BRAZIL	14,234,809
VIETNAM	15,445,812
EGYPT	16,541,142
PHILIPPINES	17,634,512
PAKISTAN	17,723,216
BANGLADESH	21,453,342
JAPAN	23,016,940
USA	32,474,518
RUSSIAN FEDERATION	32,827,525
INDONESIA	53,392,709
INDIA	131,598,984 — 97,793,741 (oral tobacco users) — 229,392,725 (all tobacco users)
CHINA	311,203,202

23

FEMALE SMOKING

"Women are taking charge of their health. And for tobacco companies, that's bad news."
—THOMAS R. FRIEDEN, NEW YORK CITY HEALTH COMMISSIONER, 2007

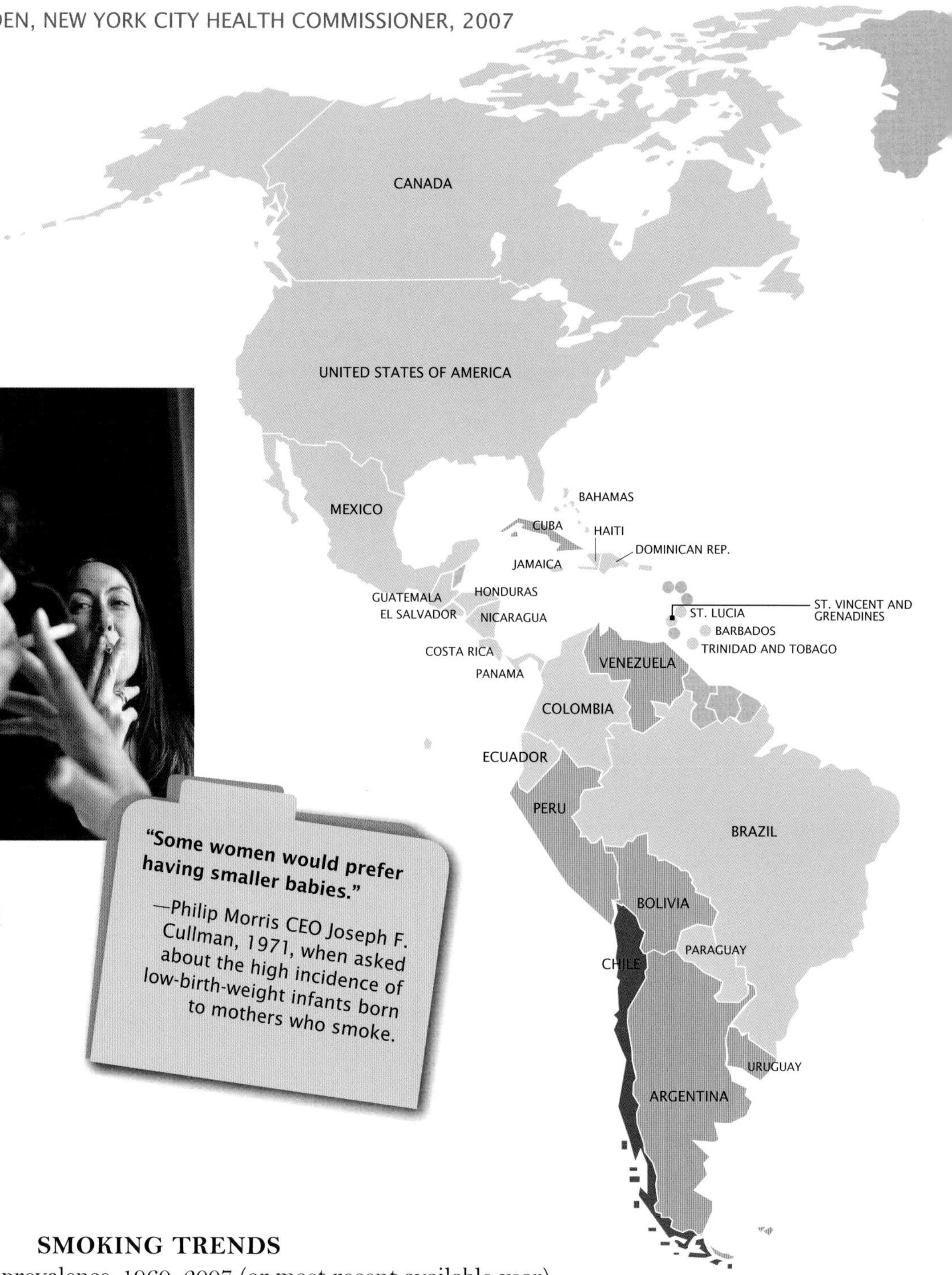

About 250 million women in the world are daily smokers; 22 percent of women in high-resource countries and 9 percent of women in low- and middle-resource countries.

Cigarette smoking among women is declining in most high-resource countries, such as Australia, Canada, the United Kingdom, and the United States, but in several southern, central, and eastern European countries, cigarette smoking rates among women are either stable or increasing.

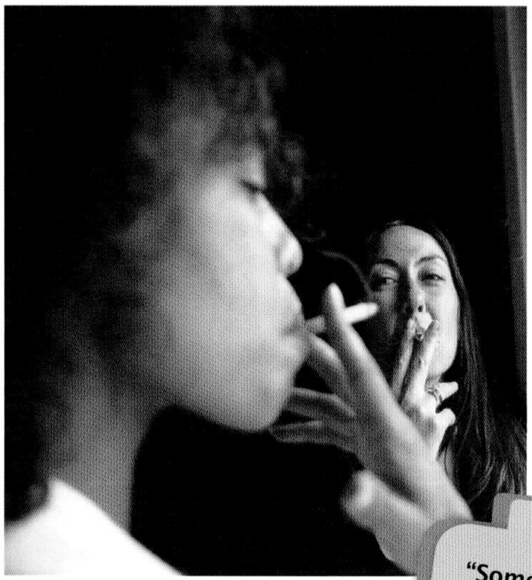

The tobacco industry markets cigarettes to women using seductive but false images of vitality, slimness, emancipation, sophistication, and sexual allure. In reality, smoking causes reproductive damage, disease, and death. Tobacco companies market a variety of cigarette brands to girls and women, including "female-only" brands that are long, extra-slim, low-tar, light-colored, mentholated, and/or candy-flavored.

If the women of the world begin smoking at the same rate as men, it will be an unmitigated global public health disaster. Preventing increases in smoking prevalence among women, especially in low- and middle-resource countries, will have a greater impact on global health than any other single intervention.

"Some women would prefer having smaller babies."

—Philip Morris CEO Joseph F. Cullman, 1971, when asked about the high incidence of low-birth-weight infants born to mothers who smoke.

CANADA

UNITED STATES OF AMERICA

MEXICO

BAHAMAS
CUBA   HAITI
JAMAICA   DOMINICAN REP.
GUATEMALA   HONDURAS
EL SALVADOR   NICARAGUA   ST. LUCIA   ST. VINCENT AND
                                                      GRENADINES
COSTA RICA   BARBADOS
PANAMA   VENEZUELA   TRINIDAD AND TOBAGO

COLOMBIA

ECUADOR

PERU   BRAZIL

BOLIVIA

CHILE   PARAGUAY

URUGUAY

ARGENTINA

SMOKING TRENDS
Adult female smoking prevalence, 1960–2007 (or most recent available year)

United States

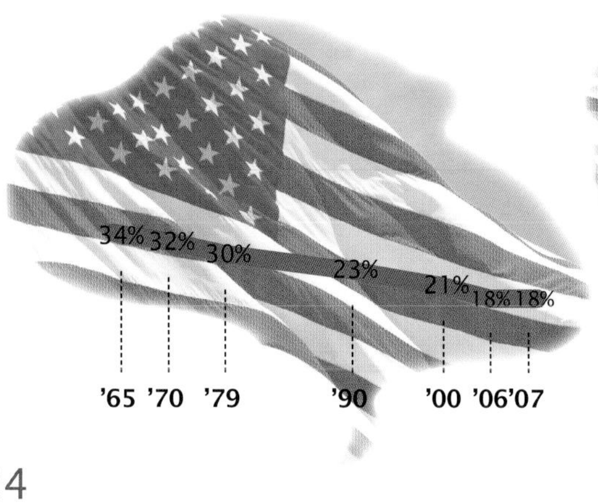

34% 32% 30%   23%   21% 18% 18%

'65 '70 '79   '90   '00 '06 '07

United Kingdom

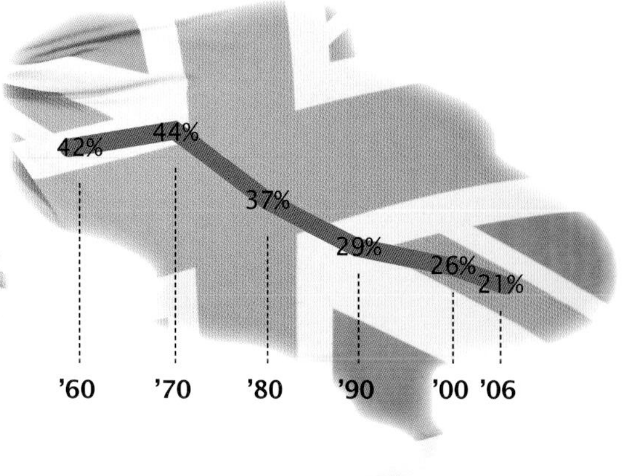

42% 44%
37%
29%   26% 21%

'60 '70 '80 '90 '00 '06

Japan

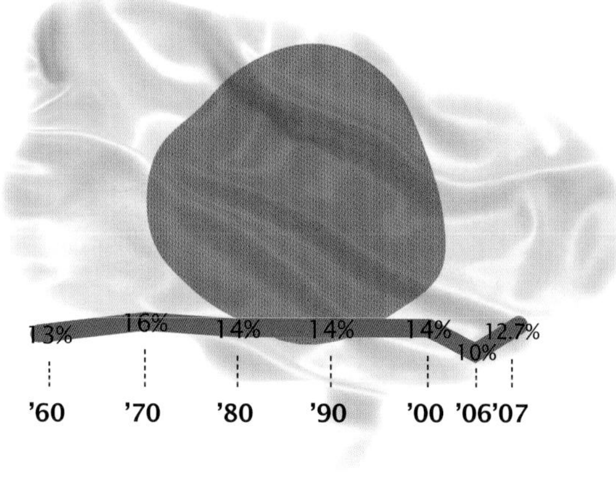

13% 16% 14% 14% 14% 10% 12.7%

'60 '70 '80 '90 '00 '06 '07

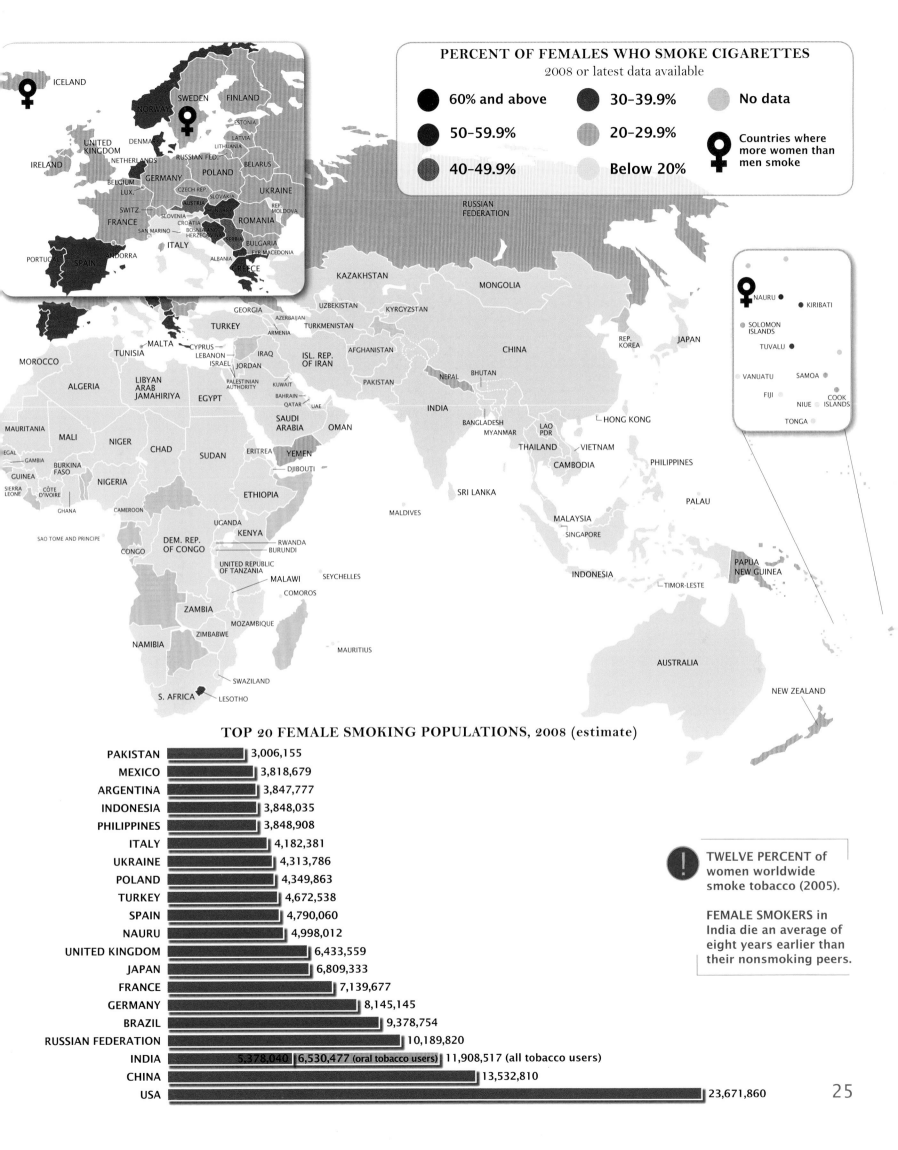

PERCENT OF FEMALES WHO SMOKE CIGARETTES
2008 or latest data available

- ● 60% and above
- ● 50–59.9%
- ● 40–49.9%
- ● 30–39.9%
- ● 20–29.9%
- ● Below 20%
- No data
- ♀ Countries where more women than men smoke

TOP 20 FEMALE SMOKING POPULATIONS, 2008 (estimate)

PAKISTAN	3,006,155
MEXICO	3,818,679
ARGENTINA	3,847,777
INDONESIA	3,848,035
PHILIPPINES	3,848,908
ITALY	4,182,381
UKRAINE	4,313,786
POLAND	4,349,863
TURKEY	4,672,538
SPAIN	4,790,060
NAURU	4,998,012
UNITED KINGDOM	6,433,559
JAPAN	6,809,333
FRANCE	7,139,677
GERMANY	8,145,145
BRAZIL	9,378,754
RUSSIAN FEDERATION	10,189,820
INDIA	5,378,040 / 6,530,477 (oral tobacco users) / 11,908,517 (all tobacco users)
CHINA	13,532,810
USA	23,671,860

TWELVE PERCENT of women worldwide smoke tobacco (2005).

FEMALE SMOKERS in India die an average of eight years earlier than their nonsmoking peers.

HEALTH PROFESSIONALS

"The role and image of the health professional are essential in promoting tobacco-free lifestyles and cultures."
—WORLD HEALTH ORGANIZATION, 2005

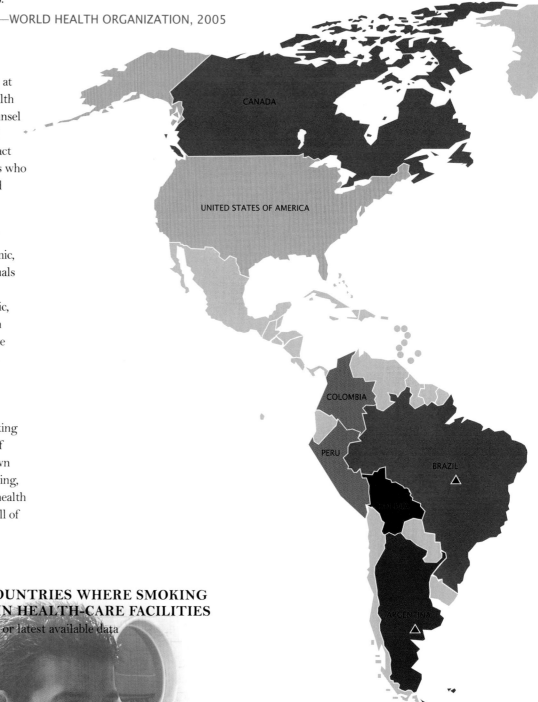

Whether in the doctor's office, the dentist's chair, at the bedside, or over the pharmacy counter, health professionals have a unique opportunity to counsel individuals about why and how to stop smoking. Even brief advice from a health professional can have a significant impact on smoking cessation success. However, health professionals who smoke are less likely to help their patients quit smoking, and their advice has diminished credibility.

Health-professional smoking prevalence varies widely around the world, reflecting socio-demographic patterns of tobacco use. In the early stages of the typical tobacco epidemic, smoking rates increase earlier among higher-status individuals and social trendsetters, such as health professionals, than among the general population. In later stages of the epidemic, health professionals—direct observers of the terrible health consequences of long-term smoking—are usually among the first to quit smoking and begin working to control tobacco. Unfortunately, student health professionals rarely receive smoking cessation counseling or formal training in the treatment of nicotine dependence.

Keeping hospitals smoke-free is crucial to reducing smoking rates among health workers and eliminating the exposure of patients and staff to secondhand smoke. By quitting their own addiction, becoming proficient at smoking cessation counseling, and engaging in social and political action against tobacco, health professionals can minimize and prevent tobacco's terrible toll of death and disability.

PERCENT OF COUNTRIES WHERE SMOKING IS PERMITTED IN HEALTH-CARE FACILITIES
2008 or latest available data

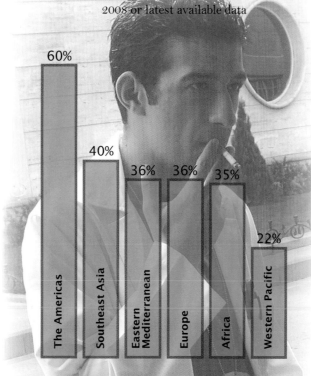

- 60% The Americas
- 40% Southeast Asia
- 36% Eastern Mediterranean
- 36% Europe
- 35% Africa
- 22% Western Pacific

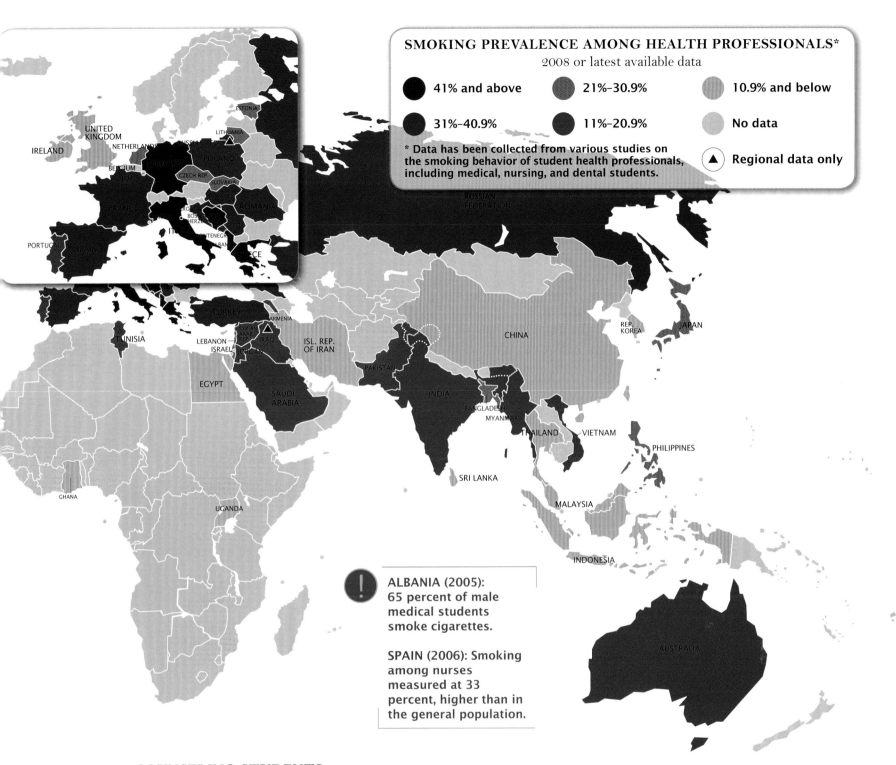

SMOKING PREVALENCE AMONG HEALTH PROFESSIONALS*
2008 or latest available data

- 41% and above
- 31%–40.9%
- 21%–30.9%
- 11%–20.9%
- 10.9% and below
- No data

* Data has been collected from various studies on the smoking behavior of student health professionals, including medical, nursing, and dental students.

▲ Regional data only

ALBANIA (2005): 65 percent of male medical students smoke cigarettes.

SPAIN (2006): Smoking among nurses measured at 33 percent, higher than in the general population.

COUNSELING STUDENTS

Percent of medical students who received formal training in smoking cessation counseling, 2007 or latest available year

Country	%	Country	%
Myanmar	43.5	Republic of Serbia	21.3
Armenia	32.3	Egypt	20.9
Iraq	31.1	Russian Federation	20.7
Syrian Arab Republic	29.3	Bolivia	20.5
Lebanon	29.1	Ghana	17.9
Vietnam	27.4	Sri Lanka	16.8
Peru	26.5	Uganda	15.9
Bangladesh	25.0	Croatia	14.5
Tunisia	24.6	Albania	10.3
Lithuania	24.2	Bosnia & Herzegovina	7.4
Nepal	23.3	Saudi Arabia	6.7
India	22.3	Argentina	5.2
Indonesia	21.8	Slovakia	3.0
Brazil	21.3	Czech Republic	1.4

"Is the physician important to P. Lorillard Company? Is the physician important to Kent?

"Indeed he is! He is the one who most frequently tells people to stop smoking . . . or to cut down on smoking."

—Lorillard Tobacco, "Kent and the Physician," confidential report, 1963

BOYS' TOBACCO USE

"Before thirty, men seek disease; after thirty, disease seeks men."
—CHINESE PROVERB

The differences in smoking rates between boys and girls are not as large as one would expect. Boys are more likely than girls to smoke, but in almost 60 percent of countries covered by the Global Youth Tobacco Survey (GYTS), there was no significant difference in smoking rates between boys and girls.

An overwhelming majority of male smokers begin using tobacco before reaching adulthood. Nearly one-quarter of young people who smoke tried their first cigarette before the age of ten.

The uptake of smoking among boys increases with tobacco industry marketing; easy access to tobacco products; low prices; peer pressure; use and approval of tobacco by peers, parents, and siblings; and the misperception that smoking enhances social popularity.

While the most serious health effects of tobacco consumption typically occur after decades of smoking, tobacco also causes immediate health effects for youth, such as reduced stamina. Young men who smoke experience significantly higher risks of erectile dysfunction than those who don't smoke, and the risk of impotence increases with every cigarette smoked.

The most important risk to adolescents is the acquisition of a life-shortening addiction. Smokers who become addicted to tobacco in their youth face the highest risks of contracting and succumbing to the most dreaded tobacco-related diseases: cancer, emphysema, stroke, and heart disease.

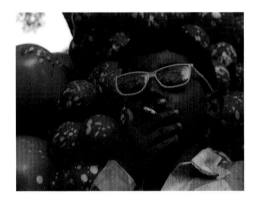

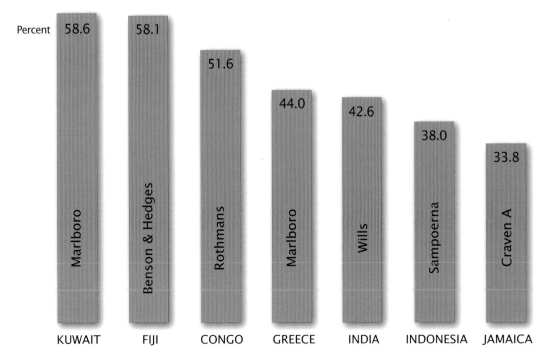

THE POWER OF BRANDING

Percent of teenage smokers who report smoking the specified brand, selected countries, 2005–2006

Brand	Percent
Marlboro (KUWAIT)	58.6
Benson & Hedges (FIJI)	58.1
Rothmans (CONGO)	51.6
Marlboro (GREECE)	44.0
Wills (INDIA)	42.6
Sampoerna (INDONESIA)	38.0
Craven A (JAMAICA)	33.8

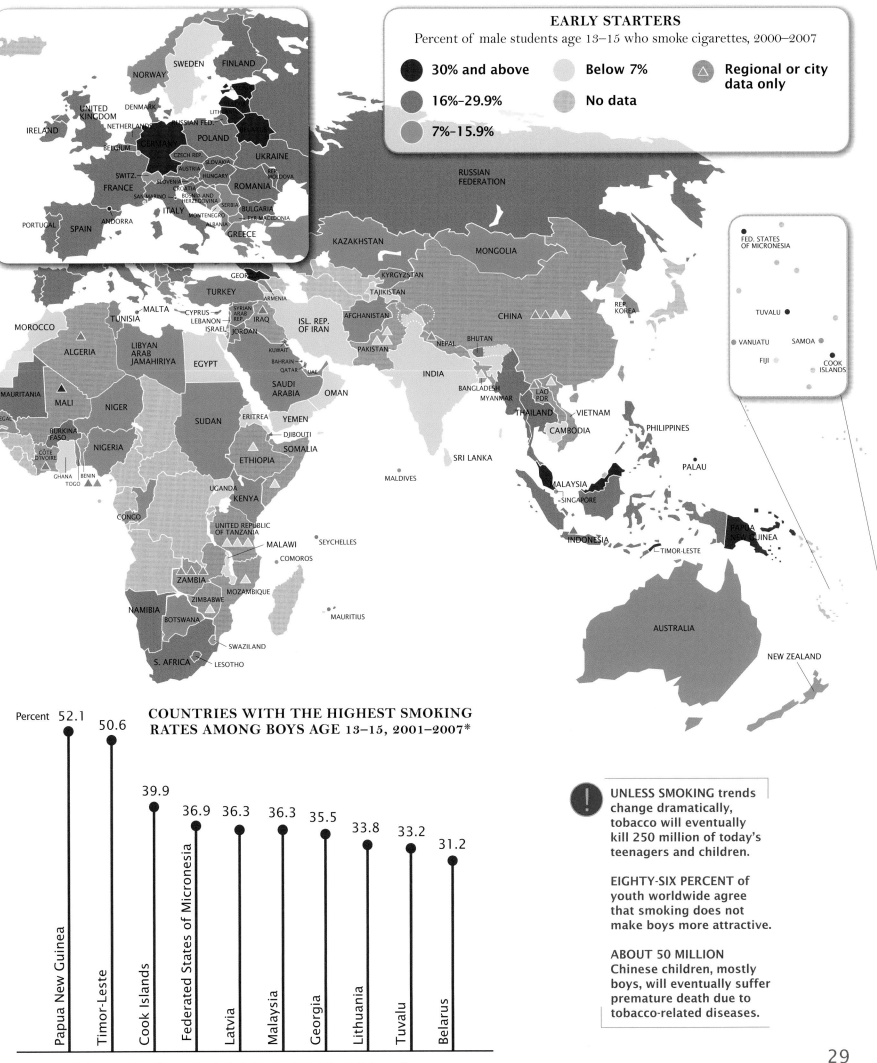

EARLY STARTERS
Percent of male students age 13–15 who smoke cigarettes, 2000–2007

- 30% and above
- 16%–29.9%
- 7%–15.9%
- Below 7%
- No data
- Regional or city data only

COUNTRIES WITH THE HIGHEST SMOKING RATES AMONG BOYS AGE 13–15, 2001–2007*

Percent

Country	Percent
Papua New Guinea	52.1
Timor-Leste	50.6
Cook Islands	39.9
Federated States of Micronesia	36.9
Latvia	36.3
Malaysia	36.3
Georgia	35.5
Lithuania	33.8
Tuvalu	33.2
Belarus	31.2

* Among selected countries included in the Global Youth Tobacco Survey

UNLESS SMOKING trends change dramatically, tobacco will eventually kill 250 million of today's teenagers and children.

EIGHTY-SIX PERCENT of youth worldwide agree that smoking does not make boys more attractive.

ABOUT 50 MILLION Chinese children, mostly boys, will eventually suffer premature death due to tobacco-related diseases.

29

CHAPTER 6

GIRLS' TOBACCO USE

Worldwide, tobacco use among girls is increasing, and the differences in smoking rates between girls and boys are not as large as one might expect. In 14 percent of countries covered by the Global Youth Tobacco Survey (GYTS), more girls than boys smoke cigarettes. Within the Western Pacific, Africa, and Eastern Mediterranean regions, boys and girls are equally likely to use tobacco products other than cigarettes. As with males, the overwhelming majority of female smokers become addicted to tobacco before reaching adulthood.

The factors that increase the risk of girls smoking are broadly similar to those of boys: tobacco industry marketing; easy access to tobacco products; low prices; peer pressure; tobacco use and approval by peers, parents, and siblings; and the misperception that smoking enhances social popularity.

In cultures where women are subjected to unrealistic body-image ideals, girls and young women may initiate smoking or rationalize their addiction in the mistaken belief that smoking assists with weight loss. In fact, cigarette smoking is not associated with a lower BMI (body mass index) in young women. Smoking prevention and cessation programs designed for girls and young women may benefit from the inclusion of counseling related to body image.

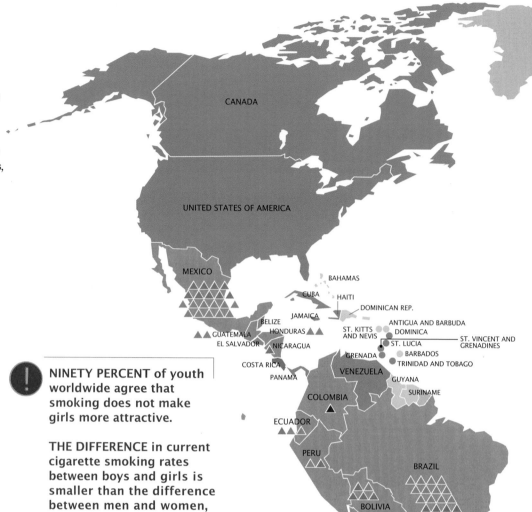

NINETY PERCENT of youth worldwide agree that smoking does not make girls more attractive.

THE DIFFERENCE in current cigarette smoking rates between boys and girls is smaller than the difference between men and women, suggesting that adult female smoking prevalence rates are likely to increase.

THE POWER OF BRANDING
Percent of teenage girls who report smoking brand as specified, selected countries, 2003–2006

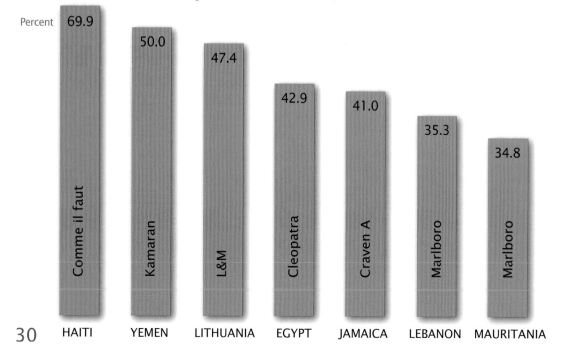

Percent						
69.9	50.0	47.4	42.9	41.0	35.3	34.8
Comme il faut	Kamaran	L&M	Cleopatra	Craven A	Marlboro	Marlboro
HAITI	YEMEN	LITHUANIA	EGYPT	JAMAICA	LEBANON	MAURITANIA

COMMON REASONS YOUNG WOMEN START SMOKING

- Global trends in women's emancipation
- Concern with weight, body image, and fashion
- Cigarette marketing campaigns targeting women
- Positive images of smoking in movies, magazines, and youth culture
- Perceived improvement in economic status
- Drug-positive subcultures

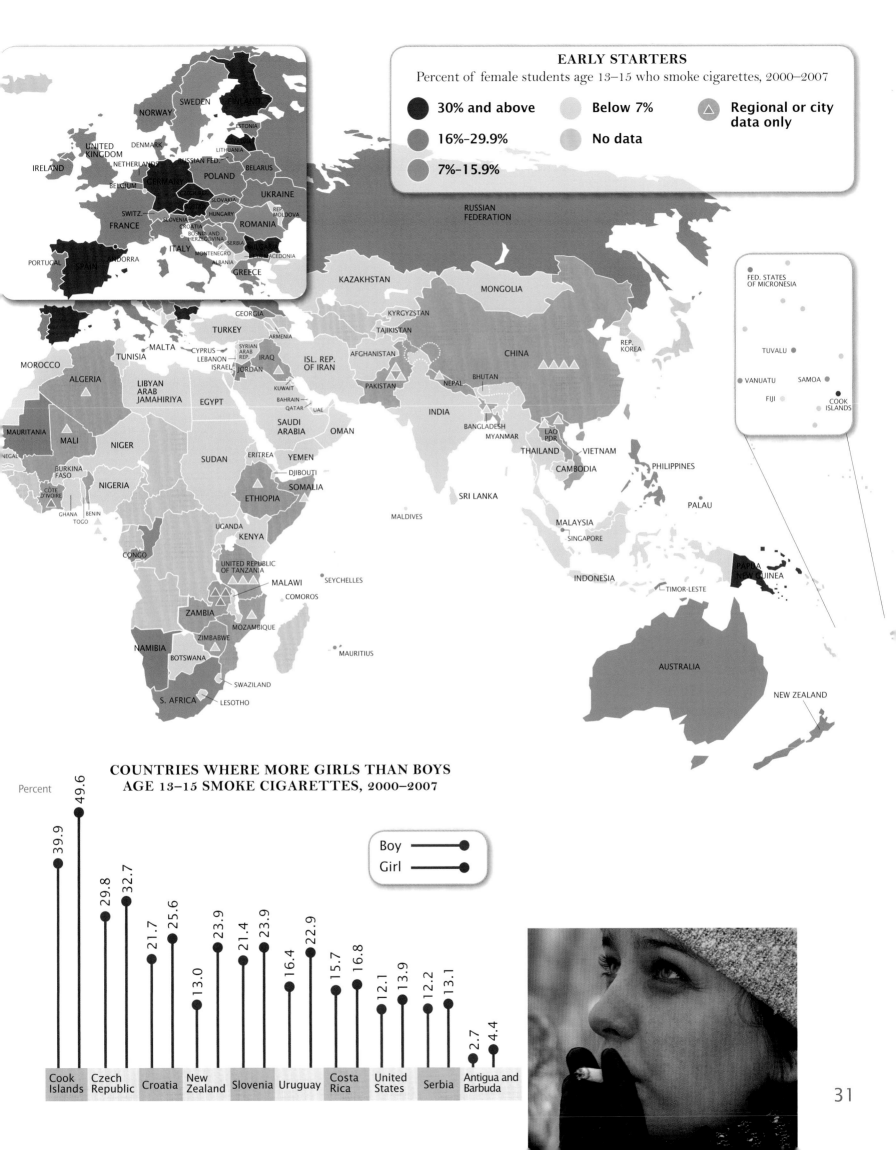

EARLY STARTERS
Percent of female students age 13–15 who smoke cigarettes, 2000–2007

- 30% and above
- 16%–29.9%
- 7%–15.9%
- Below 7%
- No data
- △ Regional or city data only

COUNTRIES WHERE MORE GIRLS THAN BOYS
AGE 13–15 SMOKE CIGARETTES, 2000–2007

Percent

Boy ———●
Girl ———●

Country	Boy	Girl
Cook Islands	39.9	49.6
Czech Republic	29.8	32.7
Croatia	21.7	25.6
New Zealand	13.0	23.9
Slovenia	21.4	23.9
Uruguay	16.4	22.9
Costa Rica	15.7	16.8
United States	12.1	13.9
Serbia	12.2	13.1
Antigua and Barbuda	2.7	4.4

31

CHAPTER 7

CIGARETTE CONSUMPTION

"China is the jewel in the crown. You could say the single biggest marketing opportunity in the world is to sell cigarettes to Chinese women."

—JEFF COLLIN, LECTURER IN INTERNATIONAL PUBLIC POLICY AT EDINBURGH UNIVERSITY, 2006

Global cigarette consumption has been rising steadily since James Bonsack invented the first cigarette-rolling machine in 1881. By the 1960s, the incontrovertible health consequences of smoking had become apparent. In some countries, consumption began leveling off and even decreasing. Worldwide, however, more people are smoking. Cigarettes account for the largest share of manufactured tobacco products (96 percent of total value sales), although in South Asia, bidi consumption exceeds cigarette consumption by an order of magnitude and use of oral tobacco remains a widespread problem.

The total number of smokers is increasing mainly due to expansion of the world's population: by 2030, the planet will support 2 billion more people than in 2000. Unless smoking prevalence rates decline dramatically, the absolute number of smokers will continue to increase. A continuing decline in male smoking prevalence may be offset, in part, by perilous increases in female smoking rates, especially in developing countries.

Unless dramatic steps are taken to control tobacco, about 6.3 trillion cigarettes will be produced in 2010—more than 900 cigarettes for every man, woman, and child on the planet. Escalating global consumption of tobacco products has created an unprecedented global public health emergency, a pandemic of epic proportions.

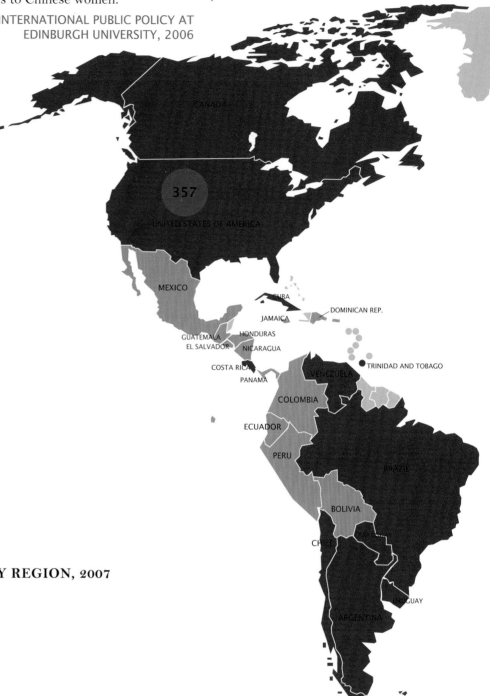

WORLD CIGARETTE CONSUMPTION BY REGION, 2007

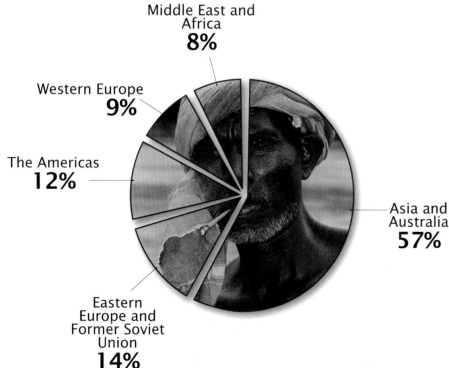

Middle East and Africa
8%

Western Europe
9%

The Americas
12%

Eastern Europe and Former Soviet Union
14%

Asia and Australia
57%

IN 2007, smokers in China consumed 37 percent of the world's cigarettes.

DURING EVERY day of the year 2010, 12 million cigarettes per minute will be smoked around the world.

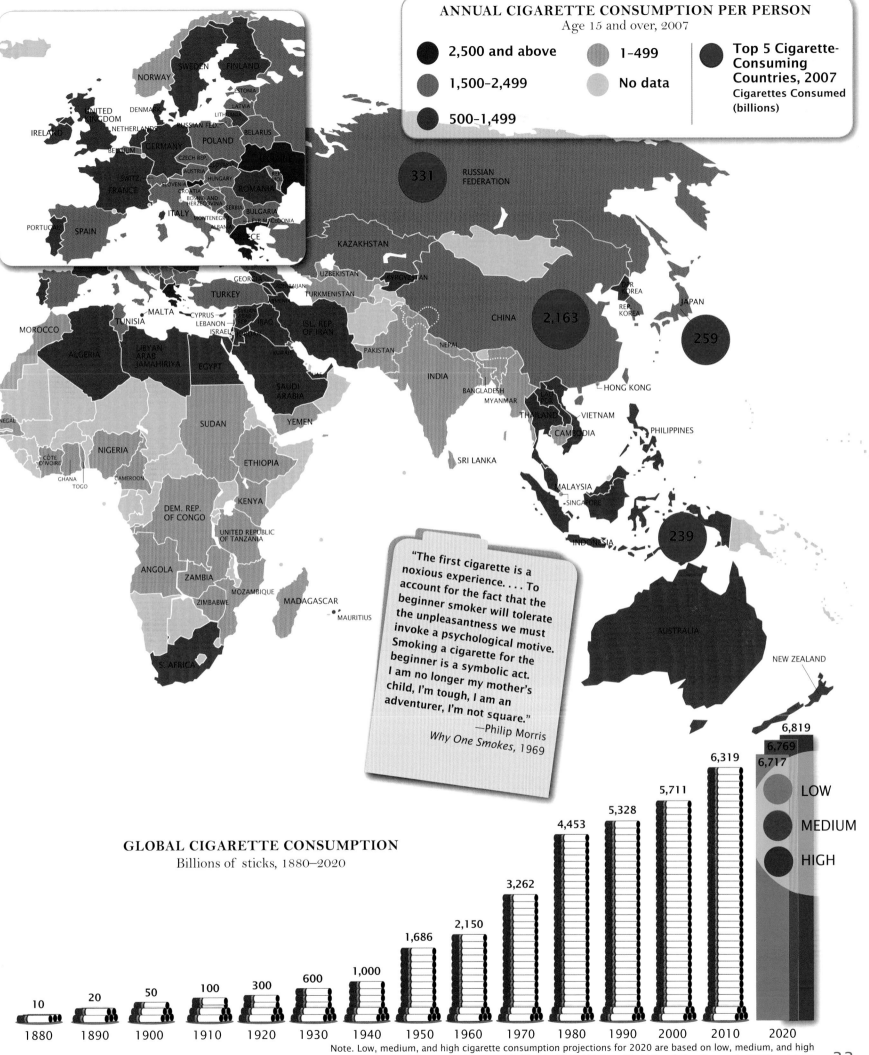

ANNUAL CIGARETTE CONSUMPTION PER PERSON
Age 15 and over, 2007

- 2,500 and above
- 1,500–2,499
- 500–1,499
- 1–499
- No data

Top 5 Cigarette-Consuming Countries, 2007
Cigarettes Consumed (billions)

RUSSIAN FEDERATION 331

CHINA 2,163

259

239

"The first cigarette is a noxious experience. . . . To account for the fact that the beginner smoker will tolerate the unpleasantness we must invoke a psychological motive. Smoking a cigarette for the beginner is a symbolic act. I am no longer my mother's child, I'm tough, I am an adventurer, I'm not square."

—Philip Morris
Why One Smokes, 1969

GLOBAL CIGARETTE CONSUMPTION
Billions of sticks, 1880–2020

Year	Value
1880	10
1890	20
1900	50
1910	100
1920	300
1930	600
1940	1,000
1950	1,686
1960	2,150
1970	3,262
1980	4,453
1990	5,328
2000	5,711
2010	6,319
2020	6,717 / 6,769 / 6,819

LOW · MEDIUM · HIGH

Note. Low, medium, and high cigarette consumption projections for 2020 are based on low, medium, and high variant population projections provided by the United Nations World Population Prospects (2000 revision).

HEALTH RISKS

"Tobacco use can kill in so many ways that it is a risk factor for six of the eight leading causes of death in the world."

—MARGARET CHAN FUNG FU-CHUN,
DIRECTOR-GENERAL, WHO, 2008

All forms of tobacco are addictive and lethal. Conclusive scientific evidence confirms that smokers face significantly elevated risks of death from numerous cancers (particularly lung cancer), heart and respiratory diseases, stroke, and many other fatal conditions. Cigar, pipe, waterpipe, and bidi smokers suffer the same types of health consequences as cigarette smokers. Cigarettes advertised as low in tar or nicotine do not reduce smoking hazards. People who chew tobacco face greatly elevated risks for cancers of the oral cavity, especially of the lip, tongue, palate, and pharynx.

Smoking and exposure to secondhand smoke impose exceptional health risks on pregnant women, infants, and children. Smoking during pregnancy is dangerous to the health of expectant mothers, potentially lethal to the fetus and infant, and may lead to lifelong health and developmental disorders among exposed children. Secondhand smoke exposure during childhood compounds the adverse health effects of fetal exposure.

Tobacco is an addictive carcinogen that directly kills half of its users, as well as nonsmoking bystanders. There is no safe form of tobacco and no safe level of exposure to secondhand smoke. However, quitting greatly reduces health risks and produces immediate and long-term health benefits. Tobacco's terrible health consequences are entirely preventable.

 PREGNANT WOMEN'S tobacco use and secondhand smoke exposure are current or emerging problems in several low- and middle-income nations, jeopardizing ongoing efforts to improve maternal and child health.

THE RISK OF dying from lung cancer is more than 23 times higher among men who smoke cigarettes, and about 13 times higher among women smokers, when compared with nonsmokers.

SMOKING SIGNIFICANTLY increases the risk of tuberculosis.

Pregnancy

HEALTH RISKS OF SMOKING DURING PREGNANCY

MOTHER

· Abruptio placentae
· Placenta praevia
· Premature rupture of membranes
· Premature birth
· Spontaneous abortion/miscarriage
· Ectopic pregnancy

FETUSES, INFANTS, CHILDREN

· Stunted gestational development
· Stillbirth
· Sudden infant death syndrome (SIDS)
· Reduced lung function and impaired lung development
· Asthma exacerbation
· Acute lower respiratory infection; bronchitis and pneumonia
· Respiratory irritation: cough, phlegm, wheeze
· Childhood cancers: leukemia, lymphoma, brain tumor
· Oral cleft

DEADLY CHEMICALS

Tobacco smoke contains more than 4,000 chemicals, more than fifty known or suspected carcinogens, and many potent irritants.

Tobacco smoke includes:	As found in:
Acetone	paint stripper
Acetylene	welding torches
Arsenic	ant poison
Benzene	Napalm
Butane	lighter fuel
Cadmium	car batteries
Carbon monoxide	car exhaust fumes
DDT	insecticide
Formaldehyde	embalming fluid
Hydrogen cyanide	capital punishment by gas
Lead	old paint, leaded gasoline
Methanol	rocket fuel
Nicotine	cockroach poison
Phenol	toilet bowl disinfectant
Polonium 210	nuclear weapons
Propylene glycol	antifreeze
Toluene	industrial solvent
Vinyl chloride	plastics

"Because known carcinogens are produced from such a wide variety of organic materials during the process of pyrolysis, it is most unlikely that a completely safe form of tobacco smoking can be evolved."

—British American Tobacco, 1965

How tobacco harms you

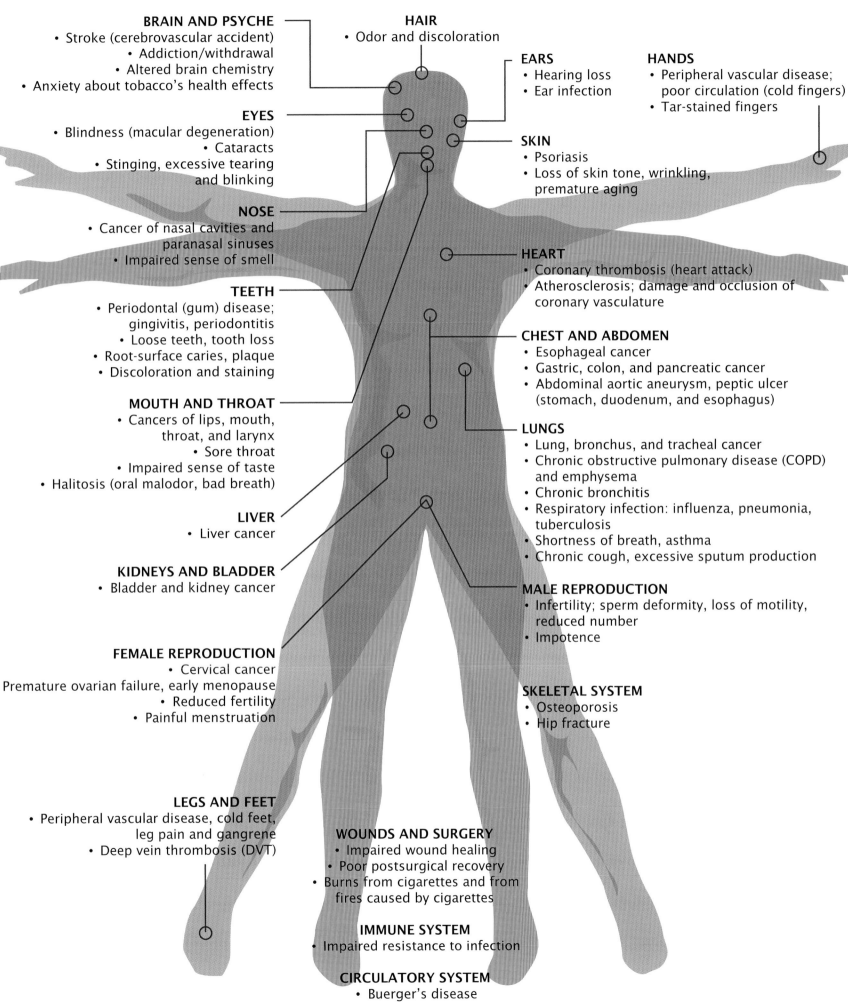

BRAIN AND PSYCHE
- Stroke (cerebrovascular accident)
- Addiction/withdrawal
- Altered brain chemistry
- Anxiety about tobacco's health effects

HAIR
- Odor and discoloration

EARS
- Hearing loss
- Ear infection

HANDS
- Peripheral vascular disease; poor circulation (cold fingers)
- Tar-stained fingers

EYES
- Blindness (macular degeneration)
- Cataracts
- Stinging, excessive tearing and blinking

SKIN
- Psoriasis
- Loss of skin tone, wrinkling, premature aging

NOSE
- Cancer of nasal cavities and paranasal sinuses
- Impaired sense of smell

HEART
- Coronary thrombosis (heart attack)
- Atherosclerosis; damage and occlusion of coronary vasculature

TEETH
- Periodontal (gum) disease; gingivitis, periodontitis
- Loose teeth, tooth loss
- Root-surface caries, plaque
- Discoloration and staining

CHEST AND ABDOMEN
- Esophageal cancer
- Gastric, colon, and pancreatic cancer
- Abdominal aortic aneurysm, peptic ulcer (stomach, duodenum, and esophagus)

MOUTH AND THROAT
- Cancers of lips, mouth, throat, and larynx
- Sore throat
- Impaired sense of taste
- Halitosis (oral malodor, bad breath)

LUNGS
- Lung, bronchus, and tracheal cancer
- Chronic obstructive pulmonary disease (COPD) and emphysema
- Chronic bronchitis
- Respiratory infection: influenza, pneumonia, tuberculosis
- Shortness of breath, asthma
- Chronic cough, excessive sputum production

LIVER
- Liver cancer

KIDNEYS AND BLADDER
- Bladder and kidney cancer

MALE REPRODUCTION
- Infertility; sperm deformity, loss of motility, reduced number
- Impotence

FEMALE REPRODUCTION
- Cervical cancer
- Premature ovarian failure, early menopause
- Reduced fertility
- Painful menstruation

SKELETAL SYSTEM
- Osteoporosis
- Hip fracture

LEGS AND FEET
- Peripheral vascular disease, cold feet, leg pain and gangrene
- Deep vein thrombosis (DVT)

WOUNDS AND SURGERY
- Impaired wound healing
- Poor postsurgical recovery
- Burns from cigarettes and from fires caused by cigarettes

IMMUNE SYSTEM
- Impaired resistance to infection

CIRCULATORY SYSTEM
- Buerger's disease
- Acute myeloid leukemia

35

CHAPTER 9

SECONDHAND SMOKING

"The evidence is now indisputable that secondhand smoke is an alarming public health hazard, responsible for thousands of premature deaths among nonsmokers each year."

—RICHARD CARMONA, U.S. SURGEON GENERAL, 2006

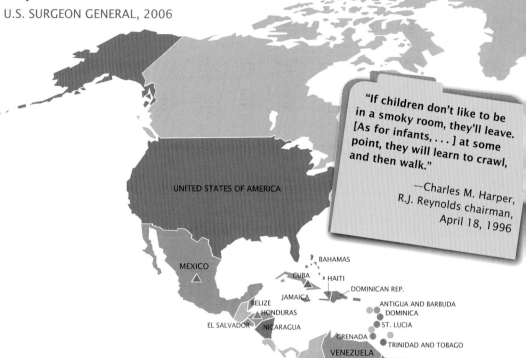

Secondhand smoke, also known as passive smoking or environmental tobacco smoke, is a mixture of sidestream smoke from the burning tip of the cigarette and mainstream smoke exhaled by the smoker. More toxic per unit of tobacco than mainstream smoke, sidestream smoke is the major component of secondhand smoke. At least fifty carcinogenic chemicals have been identified in secondhand smoke.

Nonsmokers exposed to secondhand smoke experience immediate cardiovascular and respiratory damage. Long-term effects of secondhand smoke exposure include lung cancer and coronary heart disease. Expectant mothers, fetuses, and infants exposed to secondhand smoke face higher risk of adverse health consequences.

Smoke-free policies provide protection against exposure to secondhand smoke. Today, nearly half the world's children are exposed to an unacceptable health hazard: tobacco smoke in their daily environment. To secure every child's right to a healthy future, adult smoking should be highly regulated or eliminated, especially among parents and expectant parents. Exposure to secondhand smoke remains one of the world's most critical environmental health hazards, leading all other lethal indoor air contaminants—including wood fires, asbestos particles, and radon.

"If children don't like to be in a smoky room, they'll leave. [As for infants, . . .] at some point, they will learn to crawl, and then walk."

—Charles M. Harper, R.J. Reynolds chairman, April 18, 1996

NONSMOKERS EXPOSED to secondhand smoke at home or at work increase their heart disease risk by 25 to 30 percent and lung cancer risk by at least 20 to 30 percent.

AFTER THE implementation of comprehensive smoke-free laws in New Zealand, bar patrons are exposed to 90 percent less secondhand smoke.

SMOKING IN THE home raises by 5 percent a child's probability of visiting a hospital emergency room for a respiratory illness.

THERE IS NO risk-free level of exposure to secondhand smoke. Breathing even a little secondhand smoke can be harmful to your health.

NUMBER OF DEATHS ATTRIBUTABLE TO SECONDHAND SMOKE IN THE 25 COUNTRIES OF THE EUROPEAN UNION
Major causes, 2002

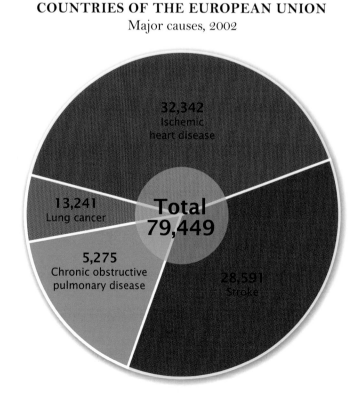

32,342 Ischemic heart disease

13,241 Lung cancer

Total 79,449

5,275 Chronic obstructive pulmonary disease

28,591 Stroke

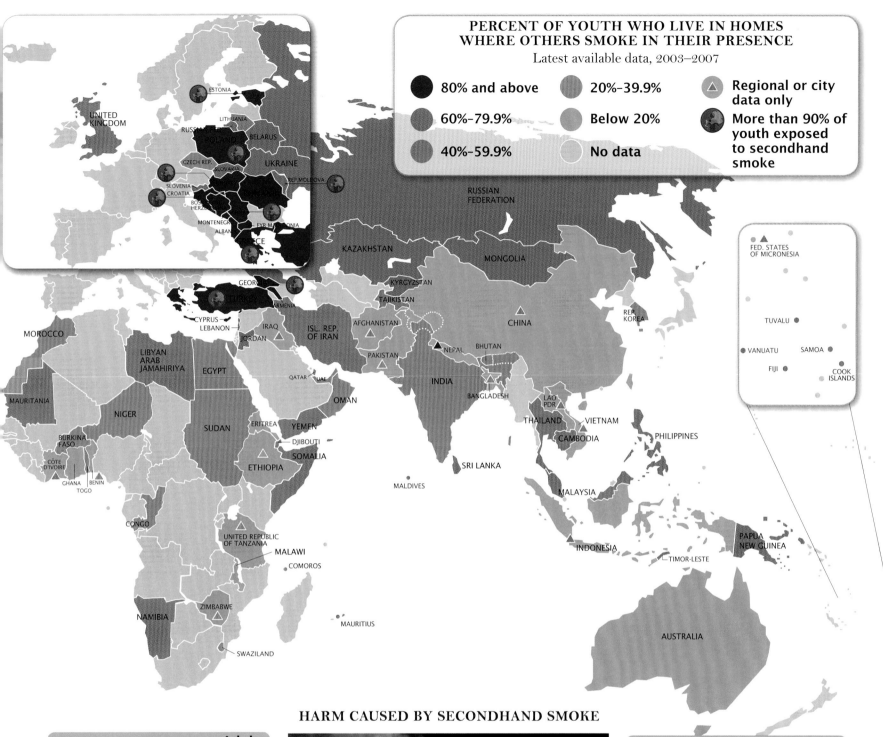

PERCENT OF YOUTH WHO LIVE IN HOMES WHERE OTHERS SMOKE IN THEIR PRESENCE
Latest available data, 2003–2007

- 80% and above
- 60%–79.9%
- 40%–59.9%
- 20%–39.9%
- Below 20%
- No data
- △ Regional or city data only
- More than 90% of youth exposed to secondhand smoke

HARM CAUSED BY SECONDHAND SMOKE

Adults

Sufficient Evidence

Coronary artery disease

Lung cancer

Reproductive effects in women

Suggestive Evidence

Stroke

Nasal sinus cancer

Breast cancer

Atherosclerosis

Chronic obstructive pulmonary disease, chronic respiratory symptoms, asthma, impaired lung function

Preterm delivery

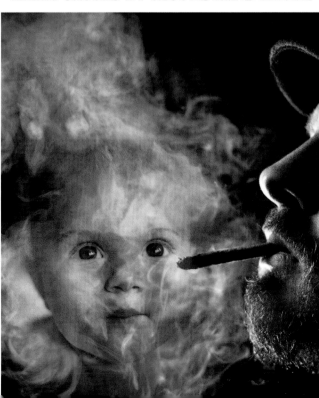

Children

Sufficient Evidence

Middle ear disease

Respiratory symptoms, e.g., cough, wheeze

Impaired lung function

SIDS (sudden infant death syndrome)

Lower respiratory illness, including infections

Low birth weight

Suggestive Evidence

Brain tumors

Lymphoma

Leukemia

Asthma

CHAPTER 10

DEATHS

"And I looked, and behold a pale horse: and his name that sat on him was Death."

—REVELATION 6:8 (KJV)

Tobacco use, in any form, is deadly. Smoking kills one-third to one-half of all lifetime users, and smokers die an average of 15 years earlier than nonsmokers. In 2010, tobacco will kill 6 million people, 72 percent of whom reside in low- and middle-income countries. If current trends continue, tobacco will kill 7 million people annually by 2020 and more than 8 million people annually by 2030.

Tobacco-attributable mortality is increasing rapidly in developing countries, and by 2030, about 83 percent of the world's tobacco deaths will occur in low- and middle-income countries. Tobacco kills more men than women worldwide because historical smoking prevalence has been higher among men than women. However, because smoking rates are increasing among women in many countries, particularly among young women, the gap in tobacco death rates between men and women is closing.

Tobacco also causes hundreds of thousands of deaths annually among nonsmokers. Occupational exposure to secondhand smoke kills 200,000 workers every year, while exposure to tobacco smoke in homes and public areas kills thousands more infants, children, fetuses, and adults. Children with developing organ systems and people with pre-existing heart and lung diseases are especially vulnerable.

One hundred million people were killed by tobacco in the 20th century. Unless effective measures are implemented to prevent young people from smoking and to help current smokers quit, tobacco will kill 1 billion people in the 21st century.

! **TOBACCO CAUSES up to 90 percent of lung cancer cases and is a major risk factor for heart attack and stroke.**

IN THE United States, secondhand smoke causes about 50,000 deaths annually.

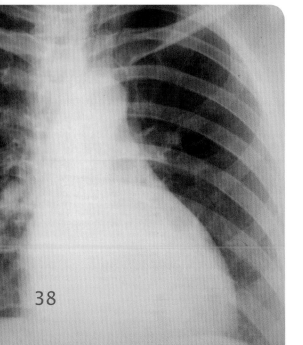

DEATHS DUE TO TOBACCO, 2015 PROJECTION

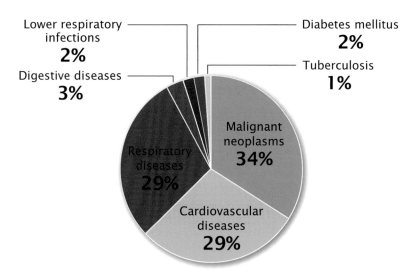

Lower respiratory infections 2%
Digestive diseases 3%
Diabetes mellitus 2%
Tuberculosis 1%
Malignant neoplasms 34%
Respiratory diseases 29%
Cardiovascular diseases 29%

PROJECTED GLOBAL TOBACCO-ATTRIBUTABLE DEATHS
By cause, 2015 baseline scenario

	Number (millions)	Percent of total
ALL CAUSES	**6.4**	**100**
Tuberculosis	**0.1**	**1**
Lower respiratory infections	**0.2**	**2**
Malignant neoplasms	**2.1**	**33**
Trachea, bronchus, lung cancers	*1.2*	*18*
Mouth and oropharynx cancers	*0.2*	*3*
Esophageal cancers	*0.2*	*3*
Stomach cancer	*0.1*	*2*
Liver cancer	*0.1*	*2*
Other malignant neoplasms	*0.3*	*5*
Diabetes mellitus	**0.1**	**2**
Cardiovascular diseases	**1.9**	**29**
Ischemic heart disease	*0.9*	*14*
Cerebrovascular disease	*0.5*	*8*
Other cardiovascular diseases	*0.2*	*4*
Respiratory diseases	**1.9**	**29**
COPD	*1.8*	*27*
Digestive diseases	**0.2**	**3**

Totals may not sum due to rounding

CUMULATIVE TOBACCO-RELATED DEATHS
Worldwide, 2005–2030

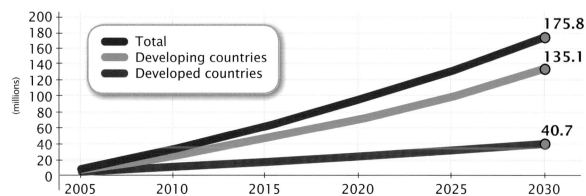

- Total — 175.8
- Developing countries — 135.1
- Developed countries — 40.7

(millions)

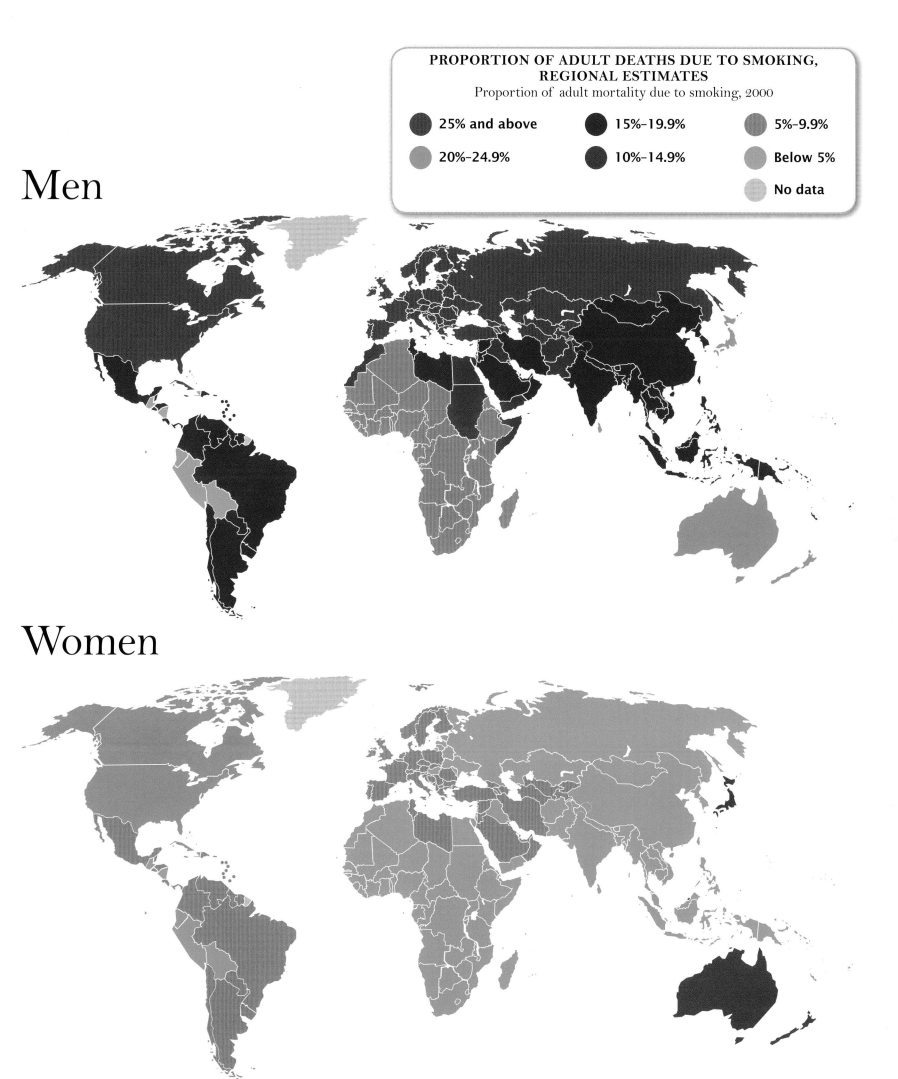

Men

Women

Proportion of adult mortality due to smoking, 2000

25% and above

20%–24.9%

15%–19.9%

10%–14.9%

5%–9.9%

Below 5%

No data

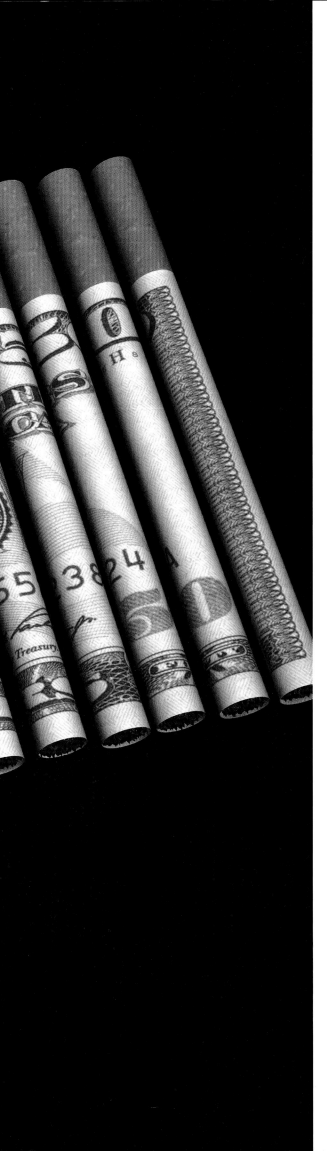

PART TWO

THE COSTS OF TOBACCO

"The super-profits of U.S. corporations are being paid for by catastrophic repercussions for the health of the younger generation."

— Gennadiy Onishchenko, Russia's chief public health officer, who instructed lawyers to explore criminal prosecution of tobacco companies for "nicotine genocide" against the Russian people.

COSTS TO THE ECONOMY

"What this case is really about is an industry…that survives, and profits, from selling a highly addictive product which causes diseases that lead to a staggering number of deaths per year, an immeasurable amount of human suffering and economic loss, and a profound burden on our national health care system."

—JUDGE GLADYS KESSLER, UNITED STATES DISTRICT COURT FOR THE DISTRICT OF COLUMBIA, AUGUST 17, 2006

Tobacco companies frequently attempt to persuade governmental authorities and the public that smoking has economic benefits. They claim that steps to reduce tobacco consumption will decrease tax revenues and increase unemployment, and even that smoking relieves an economic burden to national economies by hastening the death of dependent elderly. In fact, tobacco imposes enormous economic costs on every country. Tobacco's estimated $500 billion drain on the world economy is so large that it exceeds the total annual expenditure on health in all low- and middle-resource countries.

Tobacco's economic costs extend beyond the direct costs of tobacco-related death and related productivity losses. Other costs include health-care expenditures for active and passive smokers, employee absenteeism and reduced labor productivity, fire damage due to careless smokers, increased cleaning costs, and widespread environmental harm from large-scale deforestation, pesticide and fertilizer contamination, and discarded litter. Tobacco's total economic costs reduce national wealth in terms of gross domestic product (GDP) by as much as 3.6 percent.

Tobacco is an important cash crop in very few countries. The Framework Convention on Tobacco Control recommends that countries shift away from tobacco agriculture to economically viable alternatives. Progressive public policies encourage tobacco farmers and workers involved in cigarette manufacturing and distribution to transition into other industries that improve overall public health and welfare without sacrificing livelihoods or creating undue hardship.

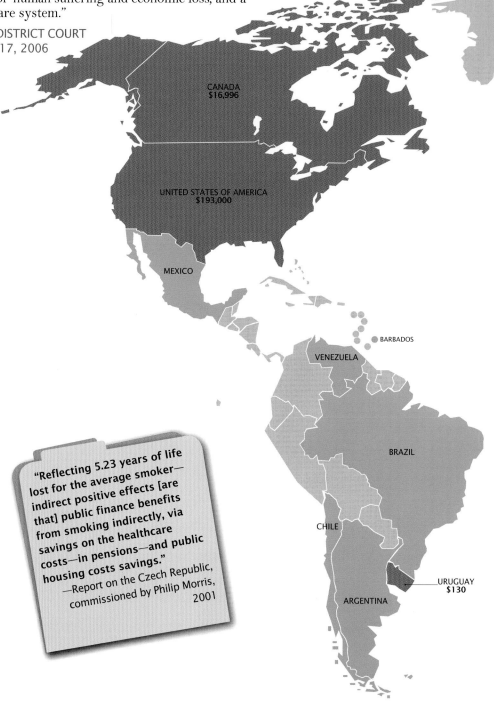

"Reflecting 5.23 years of life lost for the average smoker—indirect positive effects [are that] public finance benefits from smoking indirectly, via savings on the healthcare costs—in pensions—and public housing costs savings."
—Report on the Czech Republic, commissioned by Philip Morris, 2001

CANADA
$16,996

UNITED STATES OF AMERICA
$193,000

MEXICO

BARBADOS

VENEZUELA

BRAZIL

CHILE

URUGUAY
$130

ARGENTINA

TOTAL ECONOMIC COST OF TOBACCO AS PERCENTAGE OF GDP FOR HIGH-INCOME AND MIDDLE-INCOME COUNTRIES

2005 or latest available data

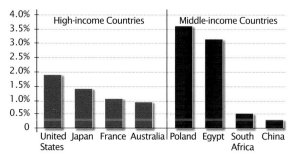

COST OF FIRES CAUSED BY SMOKING, SELECTED COUNTRIES

	United States (2005)*	Canada (2002)	United Kingdom (2005)	Japan (2003)	Worldwide (2000)**
Number of fires	82,400	7,700	3,200	3,300	1.1 million
Deaths	800	140	140	230	17,300
Injuries	1,660	470	1,100	No data	60,000
Property damage (US$)	$575 million	$84 million	No data	$89 million	$27 billion

* One-fourth of all structure fire deaths involved smoking materials / **Ten percent of all fire deaths

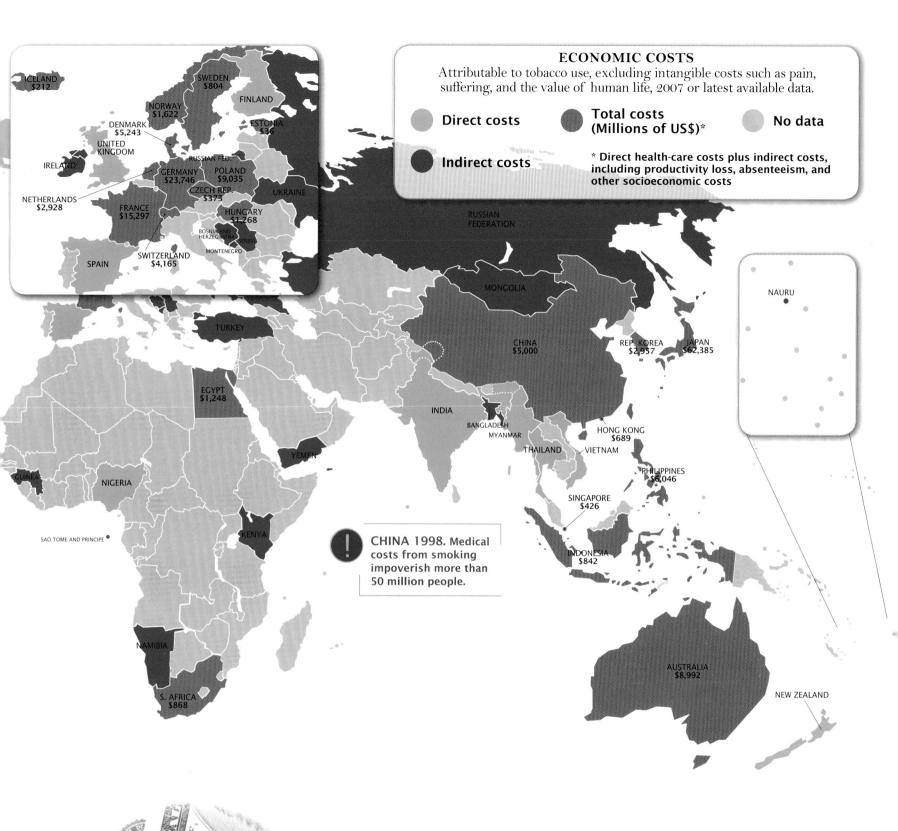

ECONOMIC COSTS

Attributable to tobacco use, excluding intangible costs such as pain, suffering, and the value of human life, 2007 or latest available data.

- Direct costs
- Indirect costs
- Total costs (Millions of US$)*
- No data

* Direct health-care costs plus indirect costs, including productivity loss, absenteeism, and other socioeconomic costs

ICELAND $212

SWEDEN $804

FINLAND

NORWAY $1,622

DENMARK $5,243

UNITED KINGDOM

ESTONIA $36

IRELAND

RUSSIAN FED.

GERMANY $23,746

POLAND $9,035

UKRAINE

NETHERLANDS $2,928

CZECH REP. $373

FRANCE $15,297

HUNGARY $1,268

BOSNIA AND HERZEGOVINA

SERBIA

SPAIN

SWITZERLAND $4,165

MONTENEGRO

RUSSIAN FEDERATION

MONGOLIA

TURKEY

CHINA $5,000

REP. KOREA $2,957

JAPAN $62,385

NAURU

EGYPT $1,248

INDIA

BANGLADESH

MYANMAR

HONG KONG $689

THAILAND

VIETNAM

PHILIPPINES $6,046

YEMEN

SINGAPORE $426

GUINEA

NIGERIA

KENYA

INDONESIA $842

SAO TOME AND PRINCIPE

(!) CHINA 1998. Medical costs from smoking impoverish more than 50 million people.

NAMIBIA

AUSTRALIA $8,992

NEW ZEALAND

S. AFRICA $868

DIRECT AND INDIRECT COSTS TO THE ECONOMY BY COUNTRY
2007 or latest available data

COUNTRY	DIRECT COSTS MILLIONS OF US$
ARGENTINA	2,200.00
BARBADOS	20.53
BRAZIL	55.56
CHILE	1,140.00
FINLAND	239.63
INDIA	7,200.00
MEXICO	627.80
MYANMAR	13.94
NEW ZEALAND	165.65
NIGERIA	590.93
SPAIN	220.62
THAILAND	977.39
UNITED KINGDOM	2,655.48
VENEZUELA	409.07
VIETNAM	77.50

COUNTRY	INDIRECT COSTS MILLIONS OF US$
BANGLADESH	652.86
BOSNIA AND HERZEGOVINA	904.00
GUINEA	293.00
IRELAND	980.06
KENYA	1,500.00
MONGOLIA	158.00
NAMIBIA	461.00
NAURU	5.10
RUSSIAN FEDERATION	24,700.00
SAO TOME AND PRINCIPE	7.50
SERBIA & MONTENEGRO	2,800.00
TURKEY	22.40
UKRAINE	3,000.00
YEMEN	1,000.00

CHAPTER 12

COSTS TO THE SMOKER

"The cost of a thing is the amount of what I will call life which is required to be exchanged for it, immediately or in the long run."
—HENRY DAVID THOREAU, 1854

Smokers spend great sums of money on a product that damages their health and financial security. These resources could be used to cover basic human needs, such as food, shelter, clothing, health care, and education. In poverty-stricken communities where food costs represent a significant portion of household budgets, expenditures on tobacco may make the difference between an adequate diet and malnutrition for the smoker's family.

Smokers and their families are exposed to severe economic losses when they become disabled or die from tobacco-related diseases. Because one-quarter of smokers die and many more become ill during their most productive years, the loss of income is substantial. In addition, family members often invest time and scarce resources to care for sick and dying smoking relatives. In many low-resource countries, hospital treatment can absorb a family's life savings, and a visit to the hospital may involve days of travel and burdensome expenses.

Smokers expose their homes and workplaces to unnecessary fire hazards, and they often pay higher premiums for health and property insurance. The largest opportunity costs of smoking exist in countries that can least afford it, exacerbating global disparities in income and health.

ALBANIA. The average smoker wastes two months' wages (US$436) per year on cigarettes.

BANGLADESH. If the average household bought food with the money normally spent on tobacco, more than 10 million people could be lifted from malnutrition and 350 children under age five could be saved each day.

INDONESIA. Paternal smoking diverts money from basic necessities to cigarettes and increases risk of child malnutrition in rural areas.

UNITED STATES OF AMERICA
MEXICO
CUBA
HAITI
DOMINICAN REP.
JAMAICA
BELIZE
HONDURAS
GUATEMALA
EL SALVADOR
NICARAGUA
COSTA RICA
PANAMA
BARBADOS
TRINIDAD AND TOBAGO
VENEZUELA
GUYANA
COLOMBIA
SURINAME
ECUADOR
PERU
BRAZIL
BOLIVIA
PARAGUAY
CHILE
URUGUAY
ARGENTINA

PRICE OF 20 MARLBORO CIGARETTES RELATIVE TO THE PRICE OF A BIG MAC, 2007

Indonesia	-47%
Mexico	-24%
Russia	-15%
Turkey	1%
Poland	2%
Japan	10%
US	49%
Germany	58%
France	80%
UK	164%

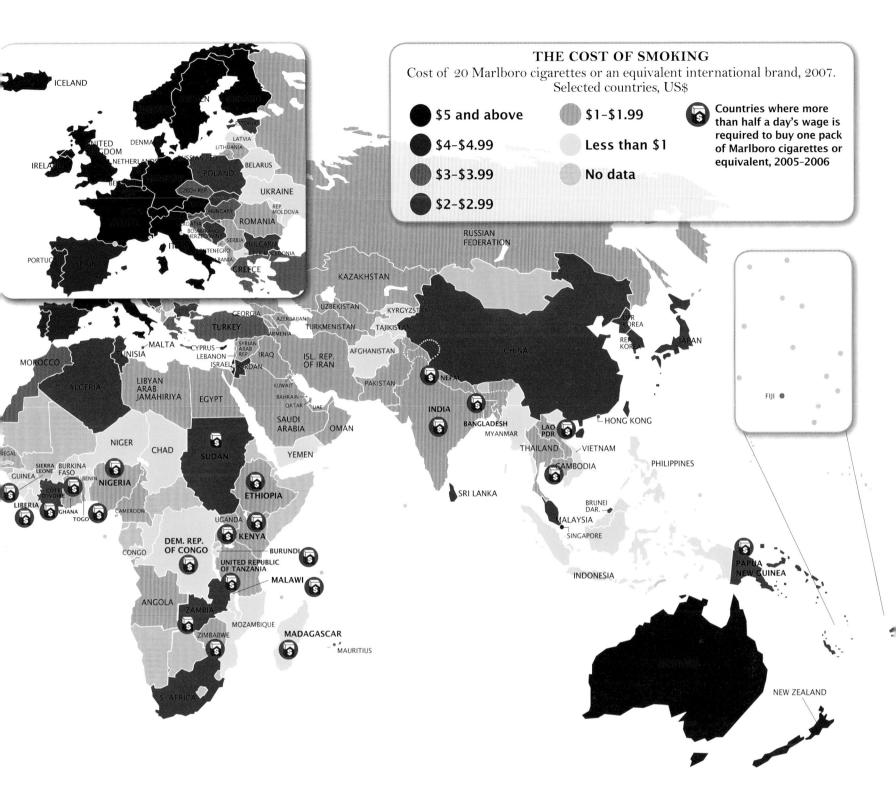

THE COST OF SMOKING

Cost of 20 Marlboro cigarettes or an equivalent international brand, 2007.
Selected countries, US$

- ● $5 and above
- ● $4–$4.99
- ● $3–$3.99
- ● $2–$2.99
- ● $1–$1.99
- ○ Less than $1
- ○ No data
- Countries where more than half a day's wage is required to buy one pack of Marlboro cigarettes or equivalent, 2005–2006

AVERAGE PRICE (IN US$) OF 1 KG OF RICE
COMPARED TO 20 MARLBORO CIGARETTES OR EQUIVALENT BRAND, 2007

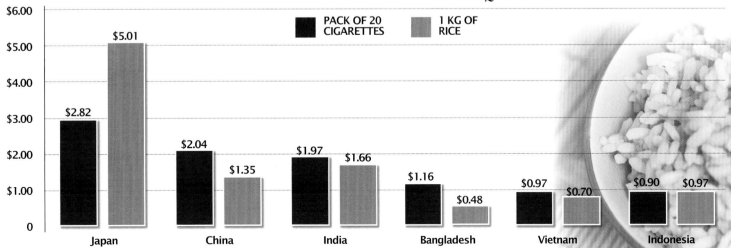

Legend:
- PACK OF 20 CIGARETTES
- 1 KG OF RICE

Country	Pack of 20 Cigarettes	1 kg of Rice
Japan	$2.82	$5.01
China	$2.04	$1.35
India	$1.97	$1.66
Bangladesh	$1.16	$0.48
Vietnam	$0.97	$0.70
Indonesia	$0.90	$0.97

45

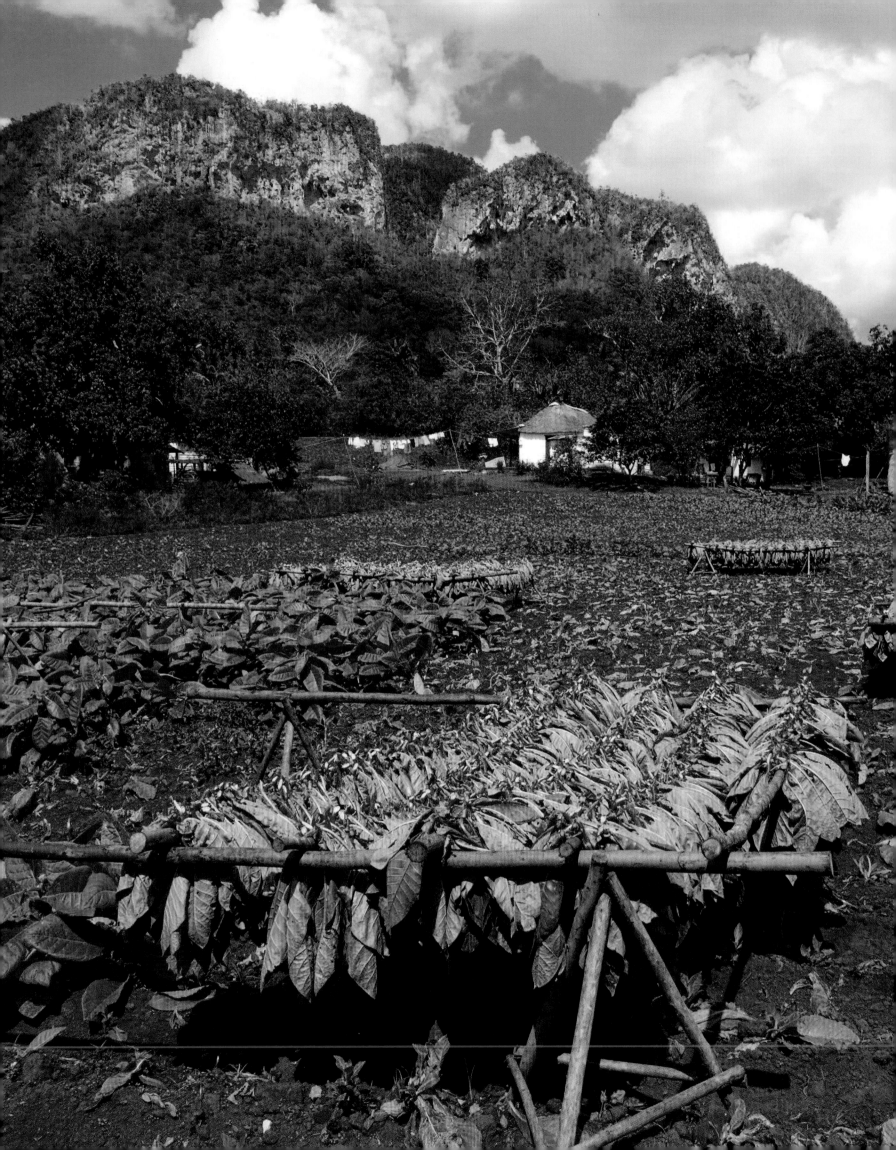

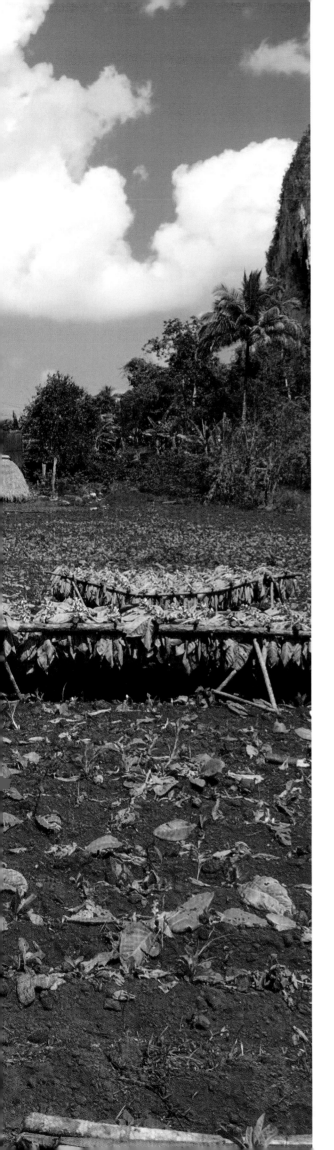

PART THREE

THE TOBACCO TRADE

"We're in a kind of business where we know that people would much rather cut down on other areas of discretionary spending before they decide to either down-trade or cut down on their overall daily cigarette consumption."

— *BAT Chairman Jan du Plessis*, Who's in the Addiction Business *(2008)*

GROWING TOBACCO

"Today, my subjects are starving and malnourished growers of tobacco, a crop
that poisons its growers, the people who handle it and all those who consume it.
. . . My subjects deserve a better livelihood than being producers of poison."

—KING SOLOMON IGURU, BUNYORO KINGDOM, UGANDA, 2004

Tobacco is grown in more than 120 countries on almost
4 million hectares of the world's agricultural land,
consuming as much arable land as all the world's
orange groves or banana plantations.

Global tobacco production has almost doubled since the
1960s, increasing 300 percent in low- and middle-resource
countries while dropping more than 50 percent in high-resource
countries. In 2006, world tobacco production totaled nearly 7
million metric tons with 85 percent of the leaf grown in low-
and middle-resource countries.

Tobacco agriculture creates extensive environmental and
public health problems. Pesticide and fertilizer runoff contami-
nate water resources, and the curing of tobacco leaf with wood
fuel leads to massive deforestation. Agricultural workers suffer
from pesticide poisoning, green tobacco sickness, and lung damage from particulate tobacco, smoke, and field dust.

Although tobacco farming is very profitable for multi-
national corporations, small farmers often fall into a debt trap
perpetuated by tobacco companies. After the cost of inputs is
deducted from revenues, small farmers often find themselves
deeper in debt.

WHO's Framework Convention on Tobacco Control calls for
financial and technical assistance to tobacco growers in countries
heavily dependent on tobacco agriculture. Shifting to nutritious,
economically viable, and environmentally sound alternatives
promises a brighter future for tobacco-producing nations.

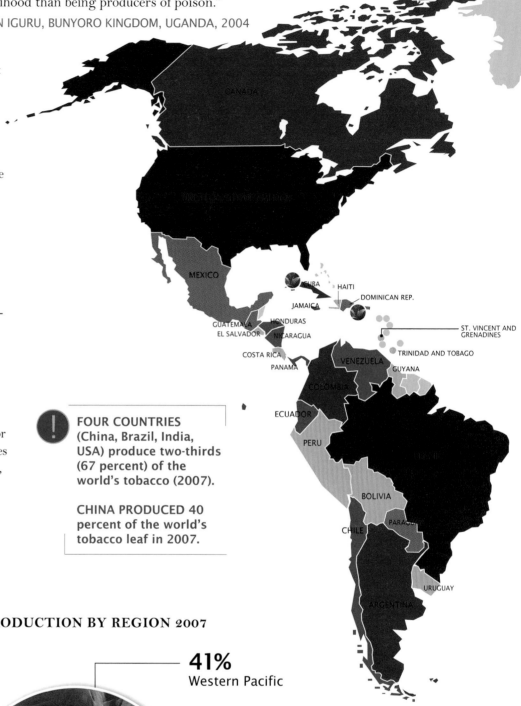

! FOUR COUNTRIES
(China, Brazil, India,
USA) produce two-thirds
(67 percent) of the
world's tobacco (2007).

CHINA PRODUCED 40
percent of the world's
tobacco leaf in 2007.

GLOBAL TOBACCO LEAF PRODUCTION BY REGION 2007

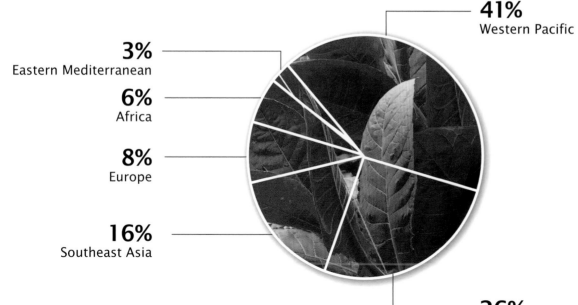

3%
Eastern Mediterranean

6%
Africa

8%
Europe

16%
Southeast Asia

41%
Western Pacific

26%
The Americas

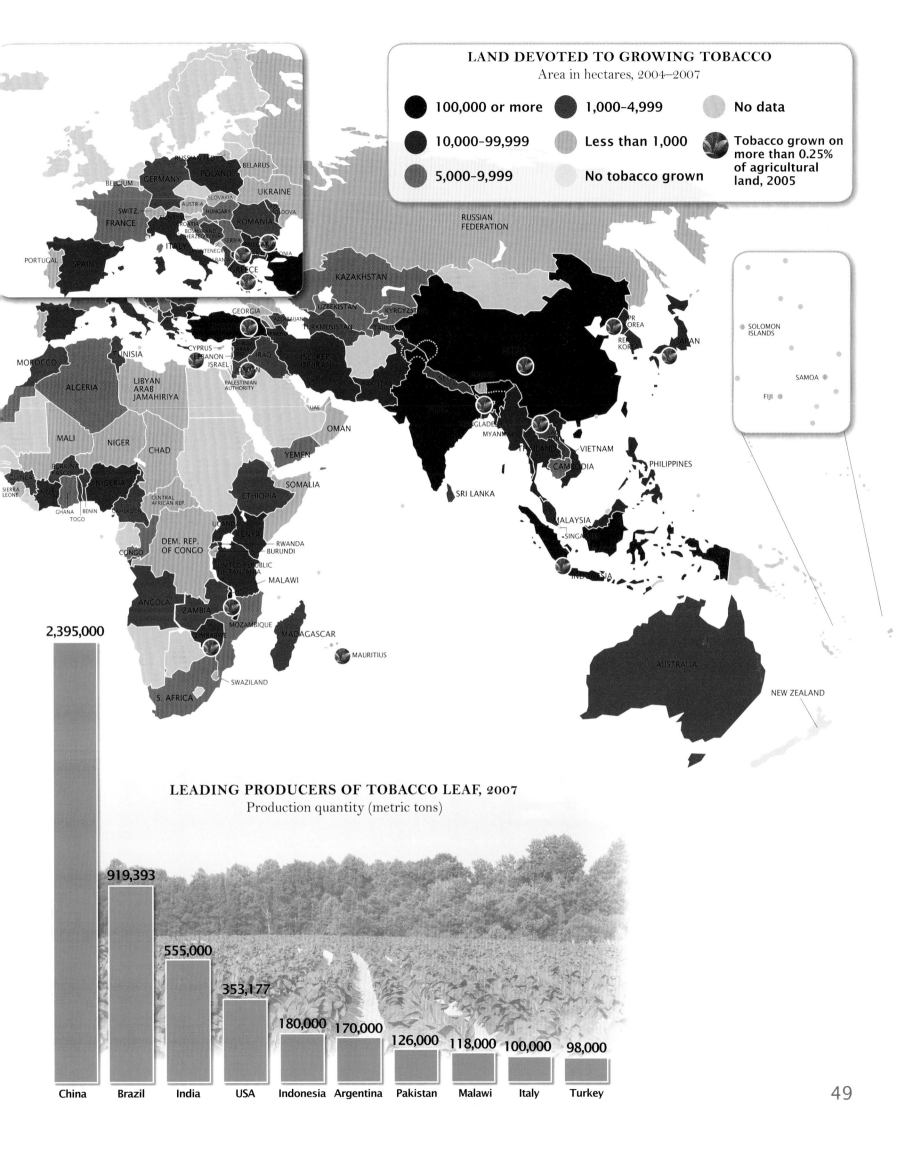

LAND DEVOTED TO GROWING TOBACCO
Area in hectares, 2004–2007

- 100,000 or more
- 10,000–99,999
- 5,000–9,999
- 1,000–4,999
- Less than 1,000
- No tobacco grown
- No data
- Tobacco grown on more than 0.25% of agricultural land, 2005

LEADING PRODUCERS OF TOBACCO LEAF, 2007
Production quantity (metric tons)

China	Brazil	India	USA	Indonesia	Argentina	Pakistan	Malawi	Italy	Turkey
2,395,000	919,393	555,000	353,177	180,000	170,000	126,000	118,000	100,000	98,000

TOBACCO COMPANIES

"In the tobacco business, big is beautiful."

—RONALD WILDMANN, AN ANALYST AT ZURICH'S BANK LEU AG,
ON THE ROTHMANS/BAT MERGER, 1999

In recent years, dozens of cigarette manufacturing companies have consolidated under four major private corporations: Altria/Philip Morris, British American Tobacco, Japan Tobacco International, and Imperial Tobacco. State monopolies are also major cigarette manufacturers. The largest state monopoly is China National Tobacco Corporation, with a global cigarette market share that exceeds that of any private company. Because the European Union intends to restrict further mergers and acquisitions that increase a tobacco company's market-share dominance, industry consolidation trends may have peaked.

The tobacco industry includes some of the most powerful transnational corporate entities in the world. Tobacco conglomerates have diversified into many other industries, such as financial services, food and beverages, pharmaceuticals, real estate, hotels, restaurants, communications, and apparel, among others. The tobacco industry is expected to continue increasing in size and power.

The global tobacco market, valued at $378 billion, grew by 4.6 percent in 2007. By the year 2012, the value of the global tobacco market is projected to increase another 23 percent, reaching $464.4 billion. If Big Tobacco were a country, it would have the 23rd-largest gross domestic product in the world, surpassing the GDP of countries like Norway and Saudi Arabia.

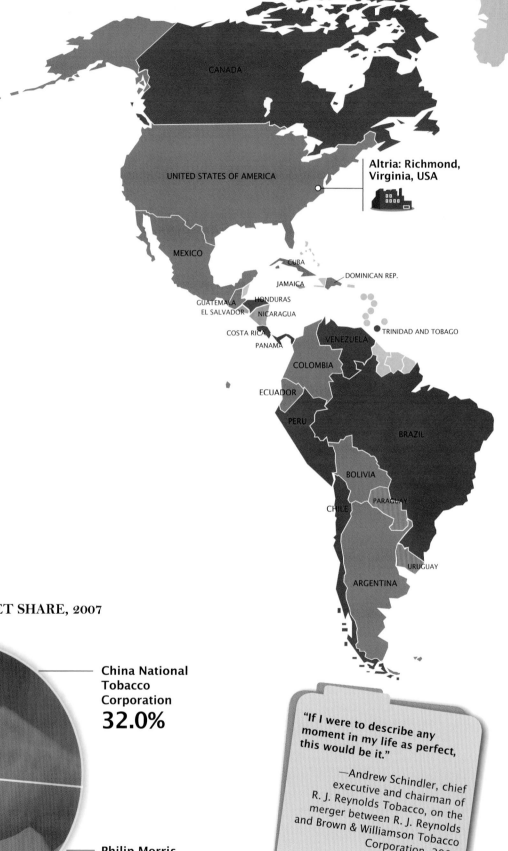

Altria: Richmond, Virginia, USA

"If I were to describe any moment in my life as perfect, this would be it."

—Andrew Schindler, chief executive and chairman of R. J. Reynolds Tobacco, on the merger between R. J. Reynolds and Brown & Williamson Tobacco Corporation, 2004

GLOBAL CIGARETTE MARKET SHARE, 2007

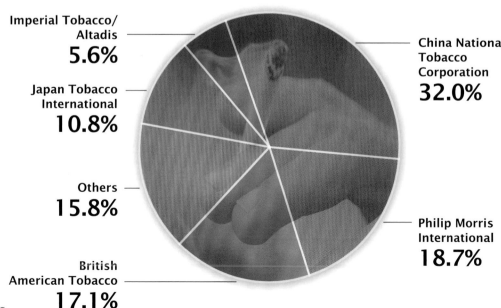

Imperial Tobacco/ Altadis
5.6%

Japan Tobacco International
10.8%

Others
15.8%

British American Tobacco
17.1%

China National Tobacco Corporation
32.0%

Philip Morris International
18.7%

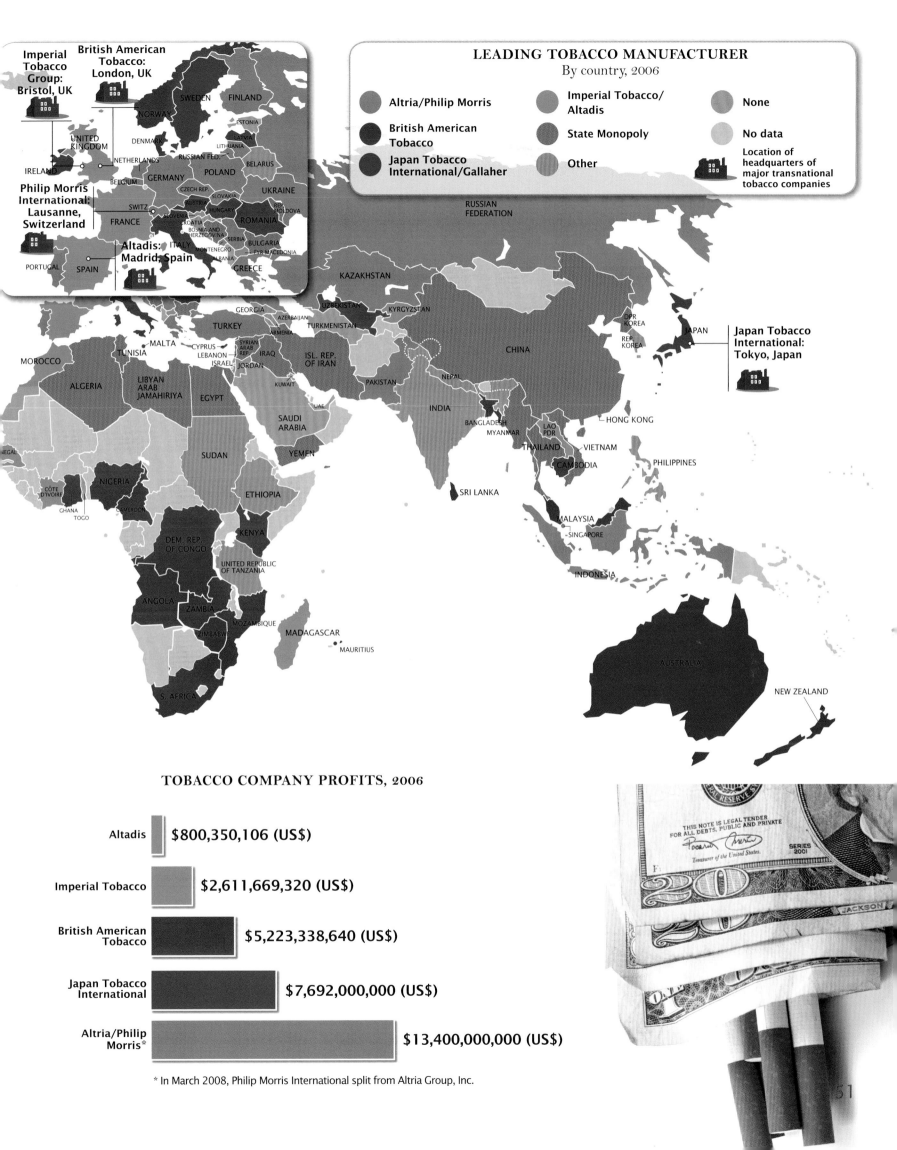

LEADING TOBACCO MANUFACTURER
By country, 2006

Imperial Tobacco Group: Bristol, UK

British American Tobacco: London, UK

Philip Morris International: Lausanne, Switzerland

Altadis: Madrid, Spain

Japan Tobacco International: Tokyo, Japan

Legend:
- Altria/Philip Morris
- British American Tobacco
- Japan Tobacco International/Gallaher
- Imperial Tobacco/Altadis
- State Monopoly
- Other
- None
- No data
- Location of headquarters of major transnational tobacco companies

TOBACCO COMPANY PROFITS, 2006

Company	Profit
Altadis	$800,350,106 (US$)
Imperial Tobacco	$2,611,669,320 (US$)
British American Tobacco	$5,223,338,640 (US$)
Japan Tobacco International	$7,692,000,000 (US$)
Altria/Philip Morris*	$13,400,000,000 (US$)

* In March 2008, Philip Morris International split from Altria Group, Inc.

51

CHAPTER 15

TOBACCO TRADE

International commodity trade in tobacco is big business, with an estimated annual value of $22 billion: $7 billion in raw material (tobacco leaves) and $15 billion in finished product (manufactured cigarettes).

China grows more than 40 percent of the world's tobacco, but only 5 percent of China's leaf is exported. Most of the remaining 95 percent is consumed domestically by China's 350 million smokers. Brazil, India, and China grow most of the world's tobacco leaf, overtaking former major producers such as the United States, where tobacco agriculture has been in steady decline for decades.

U.S. cigarette export volume has declined by more than 50 percent since 1996, valued at US$1.2 billion in 2006 (largely in sales to Japan). The Netherlands and Germany each export more than $3 billion in cigarettes annually. Many low- and middle-income countries, such as China, Malaysia, Poland, and Indonesia, are increasing capacity for cigarette production and export, competing aggressively with the major cigarette exporting nations.

To maximize profits, transnational tobacco companies seek markets with lower costs for tobacco agriculture and cigarette manufacturing, extending the tentacles of their deadly industry ever deeper into the world's nascent economies. Thwarting the tobacco industry's exploitation of emerging markets is a global health imperative.

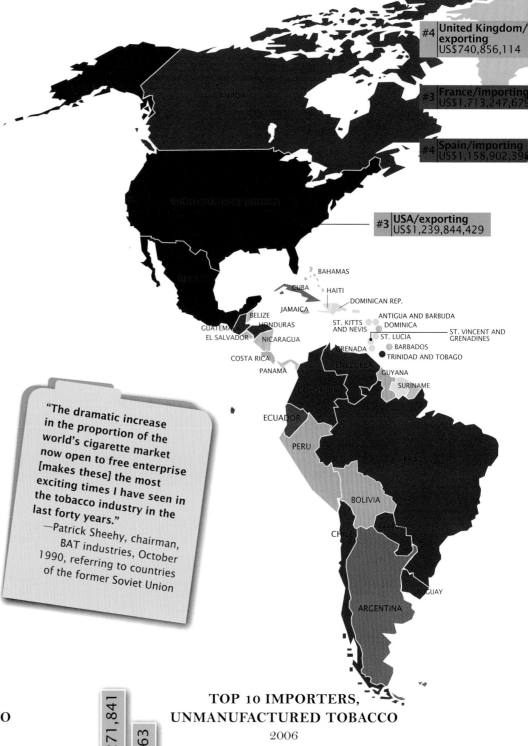

#1	Netherlands/exporting US$3,208,518,562
#4	United Kingdom/exporting US$740,856,114
#3	France/importing US$1,713,247,679
#4	Spain/importing US$1,158,902,398
#3	USA/exporting US$1,239,844,429

"The dramatic increase in the proportion of the world's cigarette market now open to free enterprise [makes these] the most exciting times I have seen in the tobacco industry in the last forty years."
—Patrick Sheehy, chairman, BAT industries, October 1990, referring to countries of the former Soviet Union

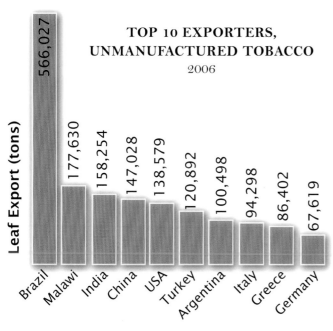

TOP 10 EXPORTERS, UNMANUFACTURED TOBACCO
2006

Leaf Export (tons)

Brazil	566,027
Malawi	177,630
India	158,254
China	147,028
USA	138,579
Turkey	120,892
Argentina	100,498
Italy	94,298
Greece	86,402
Germany	67,619

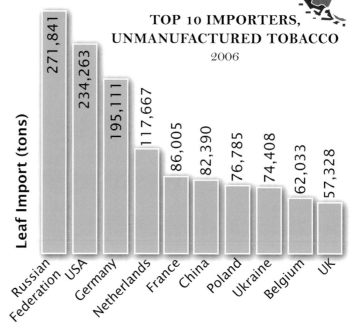

TOP 10 IMPORTERS, UNMANUFACTURED TOBACCO
2006

Leaf Import (tons)

Russian Federation	271,841
USA	234,263
Germany	195,111
Netherlands	117,667
France	86,005
China	82,390
Poland	76,785
Ukraine	74,408
Belgium	62,033
UK	57,328

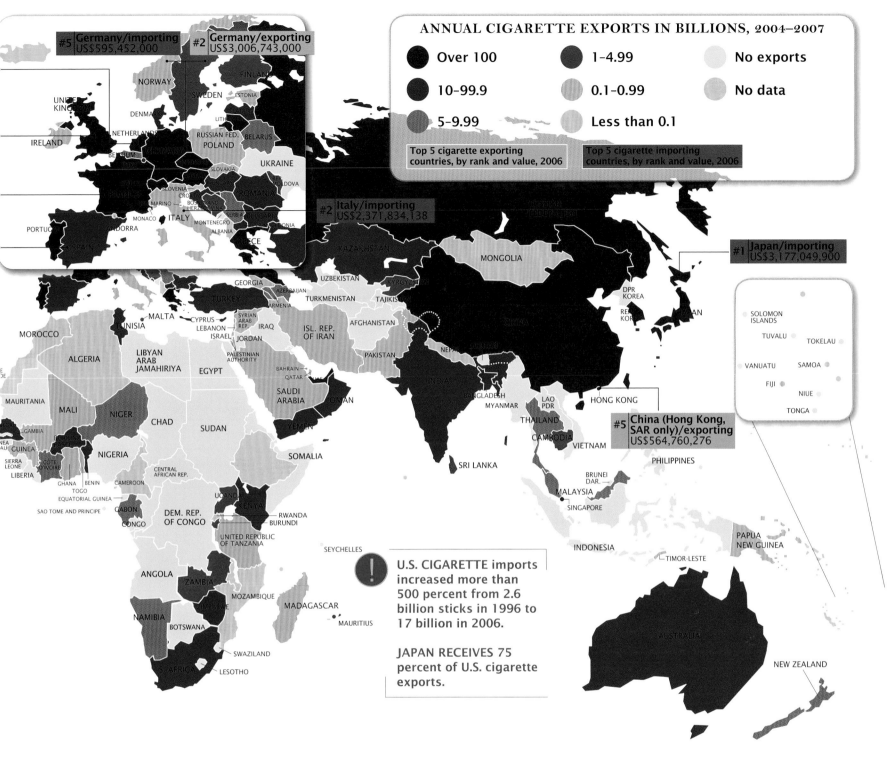

ANNUAL CIGARETTE EXPORTS IN BILLIONS, 2004–2007

- Over 100
- 10–99.9
- 5–9.99
- 1–4.99
- 0.1–0.99
- Less than 0.1
- No exports
- No data

Top 5 cigarette exporting countries, by rank and value, 2006

Top 5 cigarette importing countries, by rank and value, 2006

#5 Germany/importing US$595,452,000

#2 Germany/exporting US$3,006,743,000

#2 Italy/importing US$2,371,834,138

#1 Japan/importing US$3,177,049,900

#5 China (Hong Kong, SAR only)/exporting US$564,760,276

U.S. CIGARETTE imports increased more than 500 percent from 2.6 billion sticks in 1996 to 17 billion in 2006.

JAPAN RECEIVES 75 percent of U.S. cigarette exports.

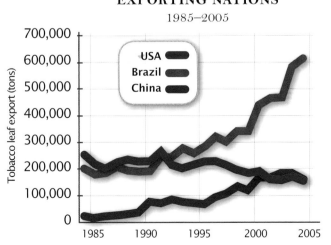

CIGARETTE EXPORT TRADE VOLUME, SELECT MAJOR EXPORTING NATIONS

1975–2005

Legend:
- USA
- Netherlands
- Germany

Y-axis: Cigarettes (billions) — 50, 100, 150, 200, 250, 300
X-axis: 1975, 1980, 1985, 1990, 1995, 2000, 2005

TOBACCO LEAF EXPORT VOLUME, SELECT MAJOR EXPORTING NATIONS

1985–2005

Legend:
- USA
- Brazil
- China

Y-axis: Tobacco leaf export (tons) — 100,000, 200,000, 300,000, 400,000, 500,000, 600,000, 700,000
X-axis: 1985, 1990, 1995, 2000, 2005

ILLEGAL CIGARETTES

"A leading international tobacco company sold large quantities of duty-not-paid cigarettes, worth billions and billions of dollars, with the knowledge that those cigarettes would be smuggled into China and other parts of the world. . . In my view, the tobacco companies were clearly putting their commercial interests above whatever moral duty they may have towards our society and to some extent such irresponsible behavior amounted to assisting criminals in transnational crime."

—JUSTICE WALLY YEUNG CHUN-KUEN, HONG KONG COURT OF APPEAL OF THE HIGH COURT, 1998

Cigarettes are the world's most widely smuggled legal consumer product. In 2006, contraband cigarettes accounted for 11 percent of global cigarette sales, or about 600 billion cigarettes. For years, the tobacco industry claimed that high cigarette taxes encouraged smuggling from low tax jurisdictions. However, documents uncovered during recent lawsuits confirm that the tobacco industry itself is responsible or involved in many large-scale cigarette smuggling operations worldwide.

Cigarette smuggling undermines public health efforts to reduce tobacco use by making international brands more affordable to low-income consumers and to youth, thus stimulating consumption. In addition, illicit products often fail to comply with health warning requirements and often violate youth access laws due to informal and underground distribution networks. Illicit trade also deprives governments of billions of dollars in annual tax revenue needed for tobacco control and to treat tobacco-related diseases. Illicit trade deprives governments of US$40–50 billion in tax revenue each year. This revenue is siphoned by organized crime networks and the tobacco companies themselves, assisting in greater sales volume and higher profit margins. Tobacco companies also smuggle cigarettes to launch new brands, enter new markets, and fight price wars with competitors.

Article 15 of the WHO Framework Convention on Tobacco Control addresses the illicit trade problem and is the basis for a new international protocol to control cigarette smuggling formulated by the parties to the Convention.

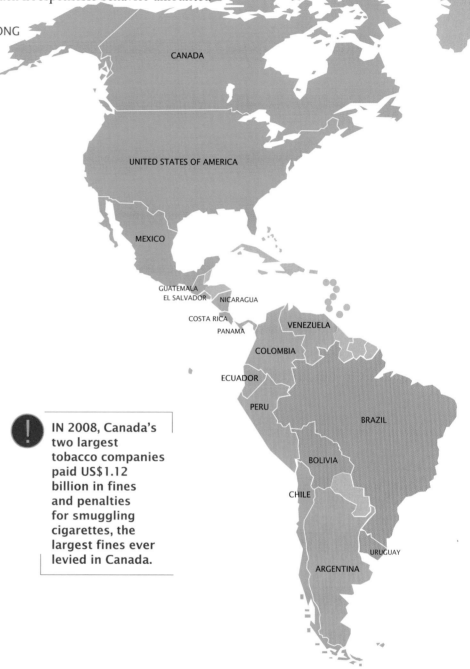

! IN 2008, Canada's two largest tobacco companies paid US$1.12 billion in fines and penalties for smuggling cigarettes, the largest fines ever levied in Canada.

SEIZURES OF CIGARETTES IN THE UNITED KINGDOM BY TYPE, 2002–2007

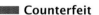

▨ **Counterfeit** ▧ **Genuine UK Brands** ▤ **Other (including non-UK brands)**

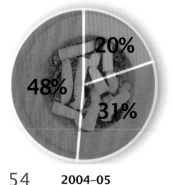

48% 20% 31%

2004–05

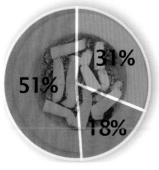

51% 31% 18%

2005–06

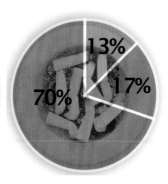

70% 13% 17%

2006–07

RECOMMENDATIONS TO CONTROL CIGARETTE SMUGGLING, FRAMEWORK CONVENTION ALLIANCE, 2007

● Track and trace tobacco products to identify points of diversion to illicit markets

● Require that cigarette manufacturers control their distribution chain, with serious penalties and tax liabilities for failure to do so

● License and monitor tobacco product supply and distribution chain personnel

● Enhance law enforcement and international cooperation to investigate and prosecute illicit trade

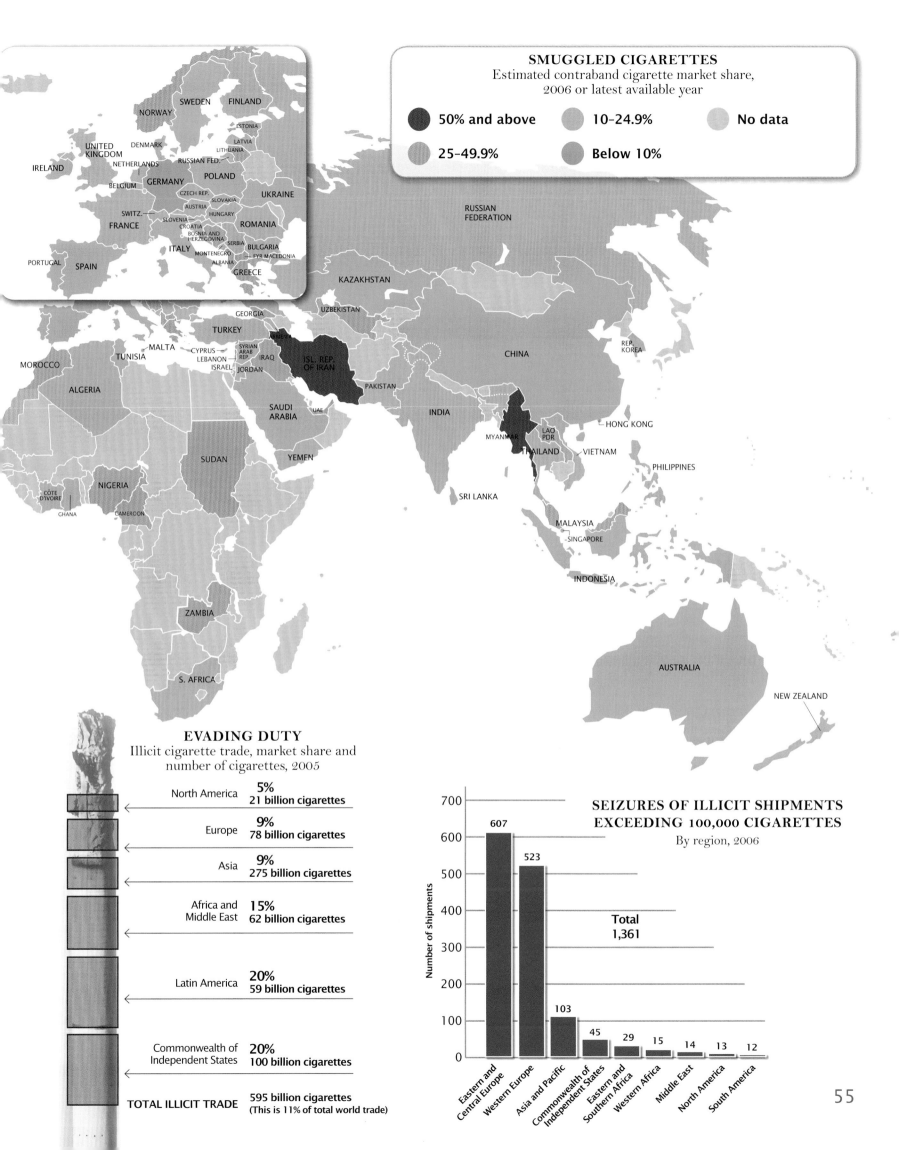

SMUGGLED CIGARETTES

Estimated contraband cigarette market share,
2006 or latest available year

- ● 50% and above
- ● 25-49.9%
- ● 10-24.9%
- ● Below 10%
- ● No data

EVADING DUTY

Illicit cigarette trade, market share and
number of cigarettes, 2005

North America	**5%**	21 billion cigarettes
Europe	**9%**	78 billion cigarettes
Asia	**9%**	275 billion cigarettes
Africa and Middle East	**15%**	62 billion cigarettes
Latin America	**20%**	59 billion cigarettes
Commonwealth of Independent States	**20%**	100 billion cigarettes

TOTAL ILLICIT TRADE   595 billion cigarettes
(This is 11% of total world trade)

SEIZURES OF ILLICIT SHIPMENTS EXCEEDING 100,000 CIGARETTES

By region, 2006

Total 1,361

Region	Number of shipments
Eastern and Central Europe	607
Western Europe	523
Asia and Pacific	103
Commonwealth of Independent States	45
Eastern and Southern Africa	29
Western Africa	15
Middle East	14
North America	13
South America	12

55

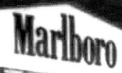

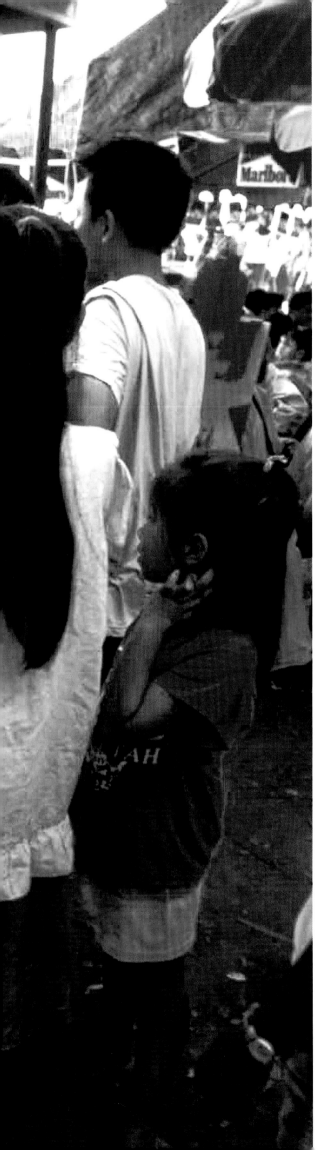

PART FOUR

PROMOTION

"You walk through there, and it makes you want to smoke. These ads are compelling even today."

— Dr. Robert Jackler, an associate dean of continuing medical education at Stanford University and curator of the tobacco ad exhibit at the NY Public Library (2008)

MARKETING

"We know that menthol cigarettes are disproportionately marketed to the African American community and that starting at a young age, menthol cigarettes are the product of choice for black smokers. . . . The industry is intentionally manipulating these products in order to get new smokers hooked."

—DR. CHERYL G. HEALTON, PRESIDENT AND CEO, THE AMERICAN LEGACY FOUNDATION, 2008

Even with increasing restrictions on marketing, tobacco companies continue to compete fiercely for cigarette market share. Between 2004 and 2007, the top-selling brand changed in more than 22 percent of the countries surveyed.

While total marketing expenditures are decreasing in the United States, companies are still spending more than $13 billion per year to encourage nonsmokers to start and to influence existing smokers to switch brands and smoke more. Tobacco companies are shifting their focus from traditional advertising to point-of-sale promotions, with 87 percent of their marketing dollars used to subsidize the price of cigarettes to encourage more consumption.

Throughout the world, tobacco companies are employing deceptive and subliminal forms of advertising, particularly through brand placement.

"We're in the cigarette business. We're not in the sports business. We use sports as an avenue for advertising our products. . . . We can go into an arena where we are marketing an event, measure sales during the event and measure sales after the event, and see an increase in sales."

— R.J. Reynolds, 1989

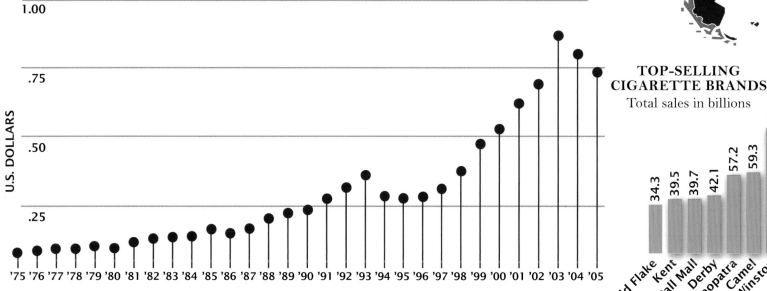

MARKETING EXPENDITURES
U.S. cigarette marketing expenditures per pack, inflation adjusted, 1975–2005

U.S. DOLLARS

1.00

.75

.50

.25

'75 '76 '77 '78 '79 '80 '81 '82 '83 '84 '85 '86 '87 '88 '89 '90 '91 '92 '93 '94 '95 '96 '97 '98 '99 '00 '01 '02 '03 '04 '05

TOP-SELLING CIGARETTE BRANDS
Total sales in billions

Wills Gold Flake	Kent	Pall Mall	Derby	Cleopatra	Camel	Winston	L&M	Mild Seven	Marlboro
34.3	39.5	39.7	42.1	57.2	59.3	91.3	106.2	111.7	472.7

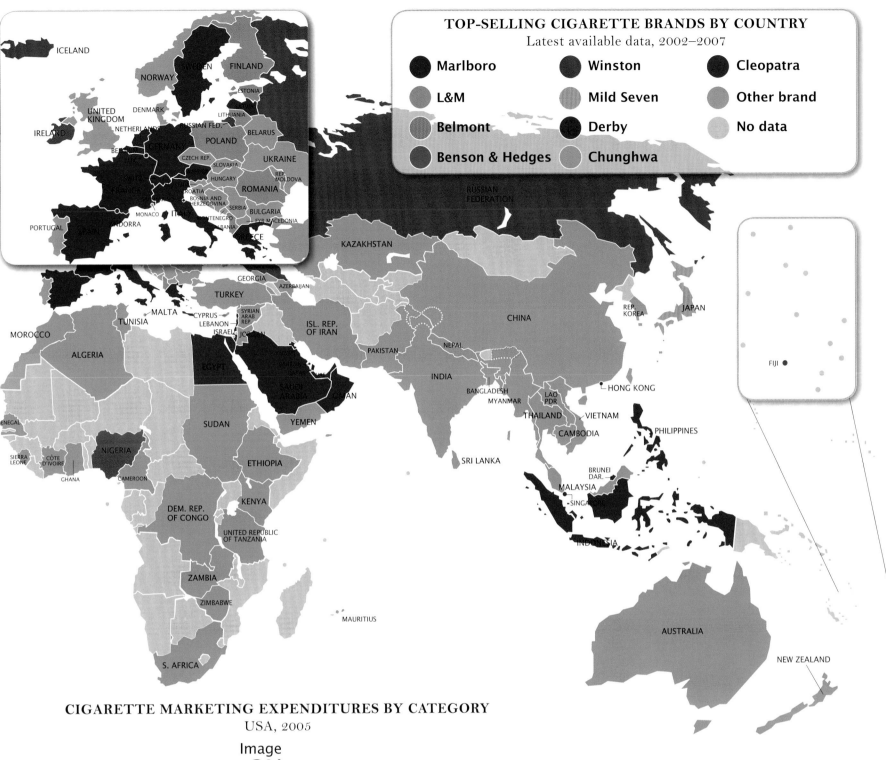

TOP-SELLING CIGARETTE BRANDS BY COUNTRY
Latest available data, 2002–2007

- Marlboro
- L&M
- Belmont
- Benson & Hedges
- Winston
- Mild Seven
- Derby
- Chunghwa
- Cleopatra
- Other brand
- No data

CIGARETTE MARKETING EXPENDITURES BY CATEGORY
USA, 2005

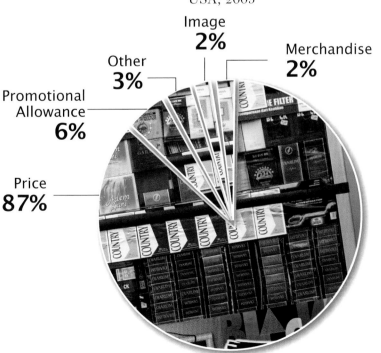

Image 2%

Other 3%

Merchandise 2%

Promotional Allowance 6%

Price 87%

BIG TOBACCO'S marketing experts and independent researchers agree: Moving stories with charismatic actors are a powerful way to attract new smokers and keep current smokers.

TODAY'S 18-YEAR-OLDS have grown up during a period in which over $100 billion has been spent to market cigarettes in the United States alone.

OF HOLLYWOOD'S top-grossing movies featuring tobacco brand placement over the past fifteen years, seven out of ten times the brand displayed is Marlboro. Studies show that brands showing up on screen most often are also the most heavily advertised in other media.

CHAPTER 18

BUYING INFLUENCE

"If you're using blood money, you need to tell people you're using blood money."

—OTIS BRAWLEY, CHIEF MEDICAL OFFICER OF THE AMERICAN CANCER SOCIETY, ON REVELATIONS THAT A TOBACCO COMPANY FUNDED LUNG CANCER RESEARCH, 2008

"The chicanery of the tobacco industry is something you almost have to admire. They are ahead of us at every turn, and they have enormous resources. . . . It's like using a muzzle-loading musket against a machine gun."

—FORMER U.S. SURGEON GENERAL C. EVERETT KOOP, 2007

The tobacco industry spends billions of dollars to influence public policy. Tobacco companies make major cash contributions to elected officials, candidates, and political parties; subsidize air travel; and finance political fundraisers, conventions, and inaugurations. Buying influence and favors through political contributions is common practice; however, most countries do not require mandatory reporting of tobacco industry inducements. In the United States, tobacco companies gave more than $34.7 million to federal candidates, political parties, and political action committees between 1997 and 2007.

To enhance their public image, tobacco companies often donate a small percentage of their profits to civic, educational, and charitable organizations worldwide. Accepting donations from tobacco companies is controversial within the academic community, and many institutions abjure it to protect their academic integrity. Tobacco companies may sponsor research, assuring complete independence, only to suppress unfavorable findings. Findings that support the tobacco industry have been published without proper disclosure of the sponsor's identity.

Despite the tobacco industry's long history of successfully buying favorable public policies and scientific research, the weight of scientific evidence and the tide of public policy continue to mount against Big Tobacco.

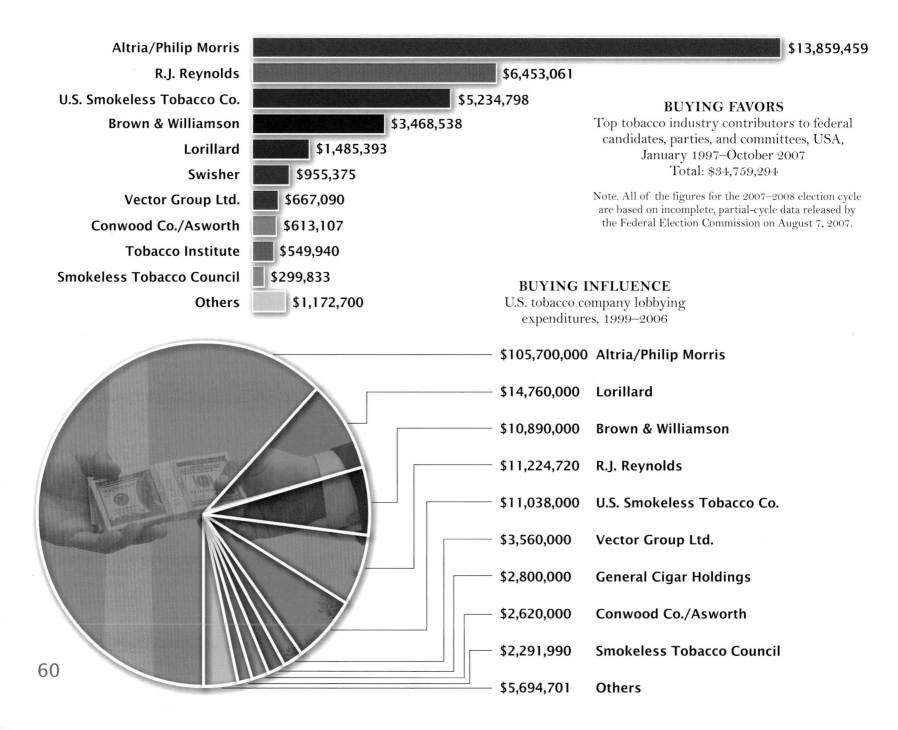

Altria/Philip Morris	$13,859,459
R.J. Reynolds	$6,453,061
U.S. Smokeless Tobacco Co.	$5,234,798
Brown & Williamson	$3,468,538
Lorillard	$1,485,393
Swisher	$955,375
Vector Group Ltd.	$667,090
Conwood Co./Asworth	$613,107
Tobacco Institute	$549,940
Smokeless Tobacco Council	$299,833
Others	$1,172,700

BUYING FAVORS
Top tobacco industry contributors to federal candidates, parties, and committees, USA, January 1997–October 2007
Total: $34,759,294

Note. All of the figures for the 2007–2008 election cycle are based on incomplete, partial-cycle data released by the Federal Election Commission on August 7, 2007.

BUYING INFLUENCE
U.S. tobacco company lobbying expenditures, 1999–2006

$105,700,000	Altria/Philip Morris
$14,760,000	Lorillard
$10,890,000	Brown & Williamson
$11,224,720	R.J. Reynolds
$11,038,000	U.S. Smokeless Tobacco Co.
$3,560,000	Vector Group Ltd.
$2,800,000	General Cigar Holdings
$2,620,000	Conwood Co./Asworth
$2,291,990	Smokeless Tobacco Council
$5,694,701	Others

Tobacco Industry Influence Exposed

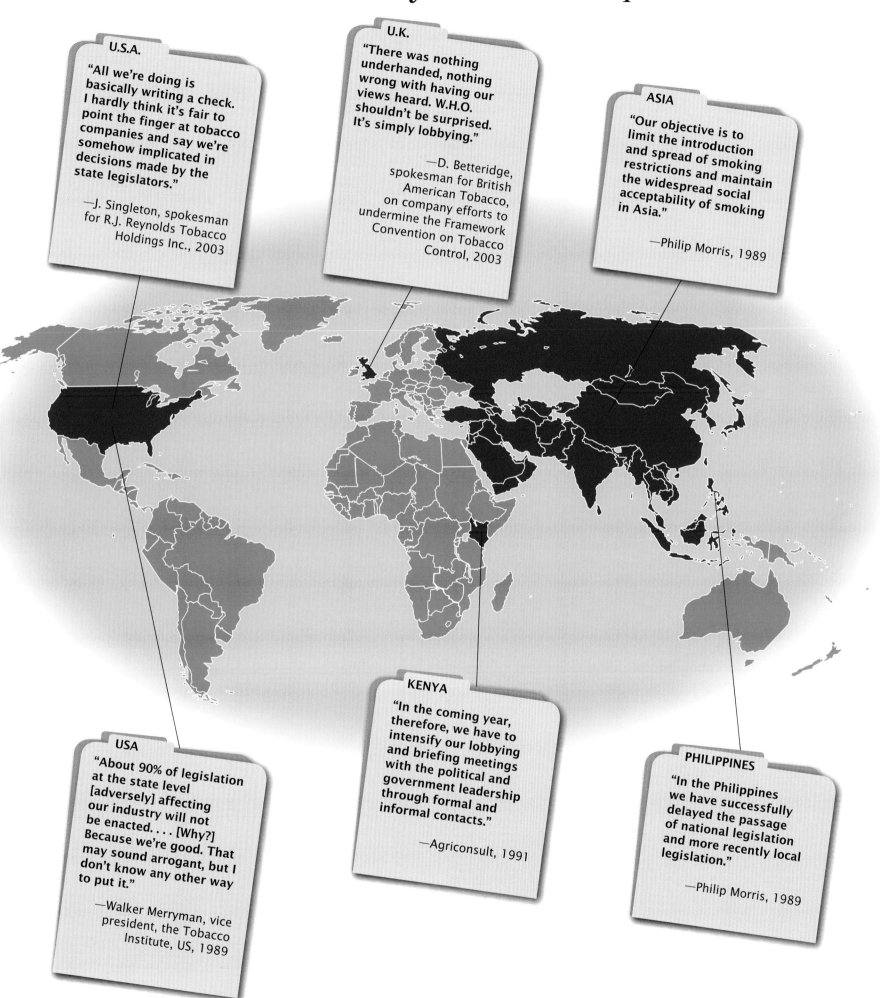

U.S.A.

"All we're doing is basically writing a check. I hardly think it's fair to point the finger at tobacco companies and say we're somehow implicated in decisions made by the state legislators."

—J. Singleton, spokesman for R.J. Reynolds Tobacco Holdings Inc., 2003

U.K.

"There was nothing underhanded, nothing wrong with having our views heard. W.H.O. shouldn't be surprised. It's simply lobbying."

—D. Betteridge, spokesman for British American Tobacco, on company efforts to undermine the Framework Convention on Tobacco Control, 2003

ASIA

"Our objective is to limit the introduction and spread of smoking restrictions and maintain the widespread social acceptability of smoking in Asia."

—Philip Morris, 1989

USA

"About 90% of legislation at the state level [adversely] affecting our industry will not be enacted. . . . [Why?] Because we're good. That may sound arrogant, but I don't know any other way to put it."

—Walker Merryman, vice president, the Tobacco Institute, US, 1989

KENYA

"In the coming year, therefore, we have to intensify our lobbying and briefing meetings with the political and government leadership through formal and informal contacts."

—Agriconsult, 1991

PHILIPPINES

"In the Philippines we have successfully delayed the passage of national legislation and more recently local legislation."

—Philip Morris, 1989

CHAPTER 19

TOBACCO INDUSTRY DOCUMENTS

"[BAT's] 'document retention' policy must be questioned. It's inconceivable that a company like this can be allowed to shred documents that can shed light on their role in Australia's number-one public health problem. These documents must have had crucial implications for public health."

—TODD HARPER, EXECUTIVE DIRECTOR OF QUIT VICTORIA, ON THE MCCABE VERDICT, 2002

Litigation against the tobacco industry has disclosed millions of secret documents containing revelations about tobacco industry conduct that have advanced tobacco control efforts around the world. Public release of these documents clearly illustrates the power of exposing tobacco industry corporate malfeasance to profoundly influence public opinion.

Under the U.S. Master Settlement Agreement, cigarette manufacturers were required to reveal internal documents and make the records available on the Internet. By U.K. court decree, BAT documents have been made publicly available at physical depositories in Guildford. U.S. documents are housed in Minnesota. Today, documents from these and other cases are available to researchers online at websites such as the Legacy Tobacco Documents Library.

The Legacy Tobacco Documents Library, supported by the American Legacy Foundation and others, is located at the University of California, San Francisco. The library contains over 8 million documents, numbering 43 million pages, providing details about tobacco industry advertising, manufacturing, marketing, sales, and scientific research.

The American Legacy Foundation grants two annual awards, one for adults and the other for youth and young adults under age 25, recognizing outstanding achievements in tobacco industry document research. Both awards honor innovative use of tobacco industry documents to achieve the primary goals of tobacco use prevention and advancement of public health.

AS OF 2008, nearly 500 research papers citing tobacco industry documents have been published.

"You can look at those documents and say maybe people made some mistakes, maybe they did some things they shouldn't have, but I don't think that shows intentional fraud. It's certainly not the conduct the companies would tolerate today."

—William Ohlemeyer, Philip Morris USA lawyer, on the Department of Justice's assemblage of incriminating documents, 2004

"In the long term, it's good for our business if fewer people get sick and die from smoking."

—Steven C. Parrish, senior vice president of Altria Group Inc., 2007

"New smokers enter the market [Nigeria] at a very early age in many cases: As young as 8 or 9 years seems to be quite common."

—Quote from "The Cigarette Market in Nigeria," 1991 BAT document discussing the habits of younger smokers in Nigeria. It is among the secret documents to be used in various Nigerian states' lawsuits.

"The situation will worsen [in Malawi] if countries fail to team up with tobacco manufacturing companies to counter the WHO anti-smoking campaign."

—Gary Faga, BAT's managing director for Malawi, on why BAT has reduced production in Malawi. The Panafrican News Agency, 2003

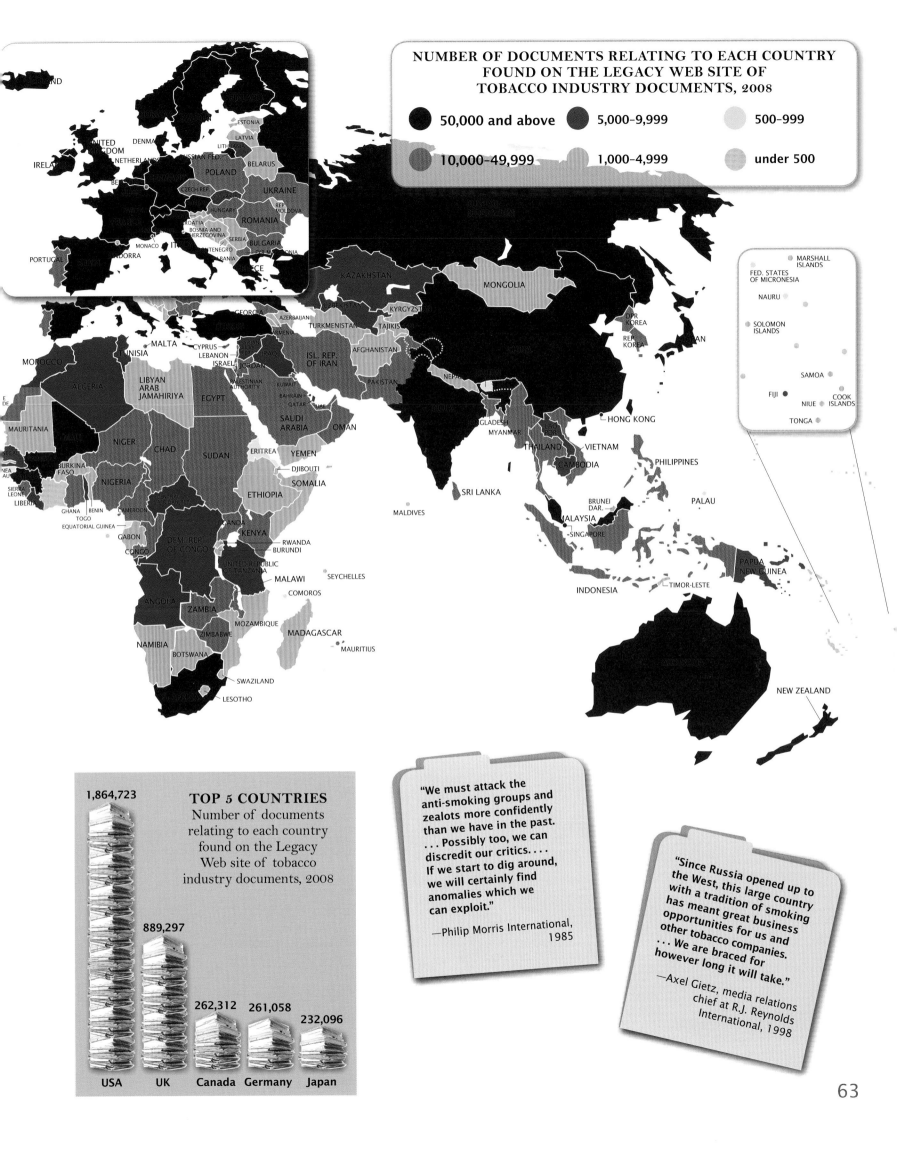

NUMBER OF DOCUMENTS RELATING TO EACH COUNTRY FOUND ON THE LEGACY WEB SITE OF TOBACCO INDUSTRY DOCUMENTS, 2008

- 50,000 and above
- 5,000–9,999
- 500–999
- 10,000–49,999
- 1,000–4,999
- under 500

TOP 5 COUNTRIES

Number of documents relating to each country found on the Legacy Web site of tobacco industry documents, 2008

1,864,723				
	889,297			
		262,312	261,058	
				232,096
USA	UK	Canada	Germany	Japan

"We must attack the anti-smoking groups and zealots more confidently than we have in the past. ... Possibly too, we can discredit our critics. ... If we start to dig around, we will certainly find anomalies which we can exploit."

—Philip Morris International, 1985

"Since Russia opened up to the West, this large country with a tradition of smoking has meant great business opportunities for us and other tobacco companies. ... We are braced for however long it will take."

—Axel Gietz, media relations chief at R.J. Reynolds International, 1998

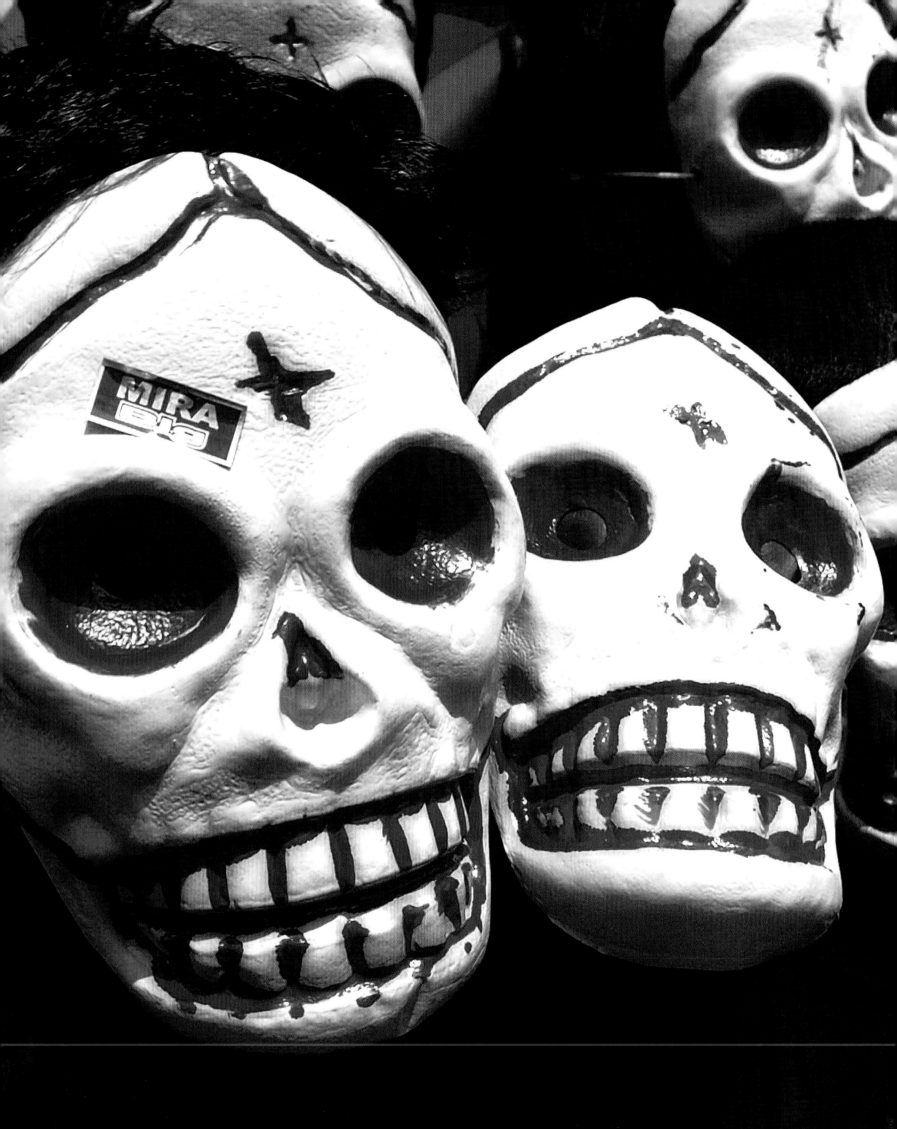

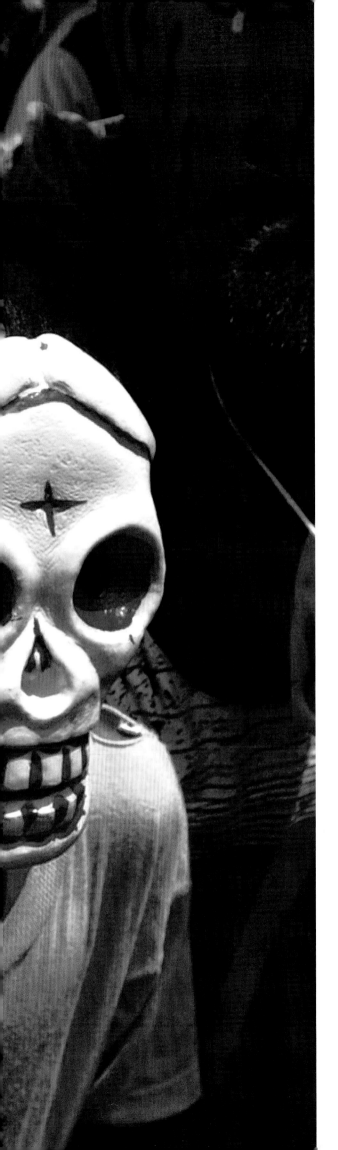

PART FIVE

TAKING ACTION

"Half measures are not enough. When one form of advertising is banned, the tobacco industry simply shifts its vast resources to another channel. We urge governments to impose a complete ban to break the tobacco marketing net."

— Dr. Douglas Bettcher, Director of WHO's Tobacco Free Initiative, which has issued a call for a worldwide ban on all tobacco advertising, promotions, and sponsorship, 2008.

CHAPTER 20

RESEARCH

"The future of tobacco control will never rest solely on the development of new research-based knowledge; it never has. Almost certainly the future will depend far more on effective politics and activism."

—KENNETH E. WARNER, PHD, DEAN OF THE SCHOOL OF PUBLIC HEALTH, UNIVERSITY OF MICHIGAN, USA

Since the 1950s, scientific research has proven the unparalleled harm tobacco causes to human health.

From high-income countries and an increasing number of low- and middle-income countries, scientific evidence has accumulated on tobacco use, the harm it causes, and actions needed to discourage its use. Barriers that make it difficult for developing countries to participate include the lack of standardized data and inadequate communication networks, tobacco-control research capacity, and human and financial resources. Despite philanthropic efforts, tobacco control research continues to be underfunded throughout the world.

Conflicts of interest in tobacco control research arise repeatedly due to the shortage of nonprofit and public-sector research funding. When tobacco companies invest resources in research, they often expect to play a role in designing, conducting, and reporting study results. To maintain the integrity of scientific research and to avoid the appearance of bias, an increasing number of researchers and institutions are unwilling to accept money from the tobacco industry. Among research funding agencies, the American Cancer Society, the National Cancer Institute of Canada, the National Heart Foundation of Australia, and members of the Association of European Cancer Leagues prohibit grants to researchers who have received support from the tobacco industry.

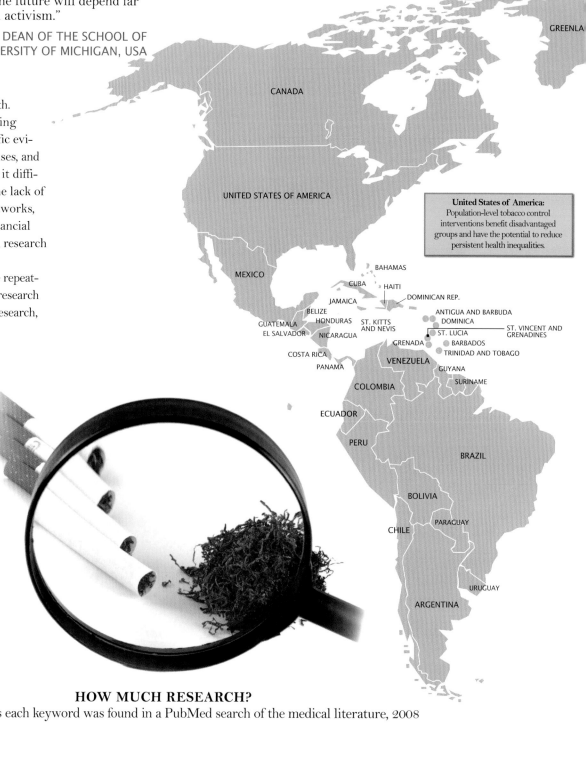

United States of America:
Population-level tobacco control interventions benefit disadvantaged groups and have the potential to reduce persistent health inequalities.

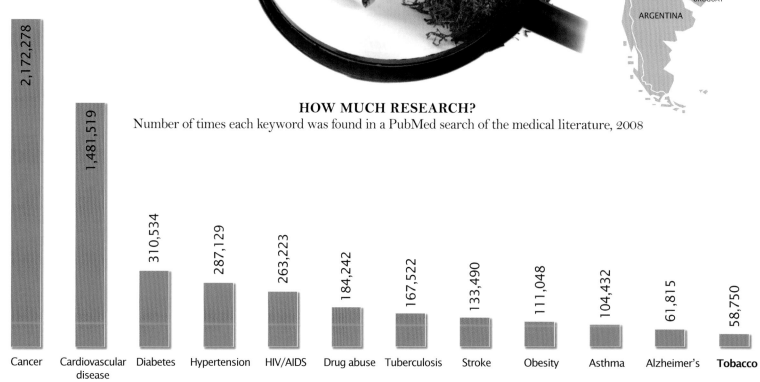

HOW MUCH RESEARCH?
Number of times each keyword was found in a PubMed search of the medical literature, 2008

Cancer	2,172,278
Cardiovascular disease	1,481,519
Diabetes	310,534
Hypertension	287,129
HIV/AIDS	263,223
Drug abuse	184,242
Tuberculosis	167,522
Stroke	133,490
Obesity	111,048
Asthma	104,432
Alzheimer's	61,815
Tobacco	58,750

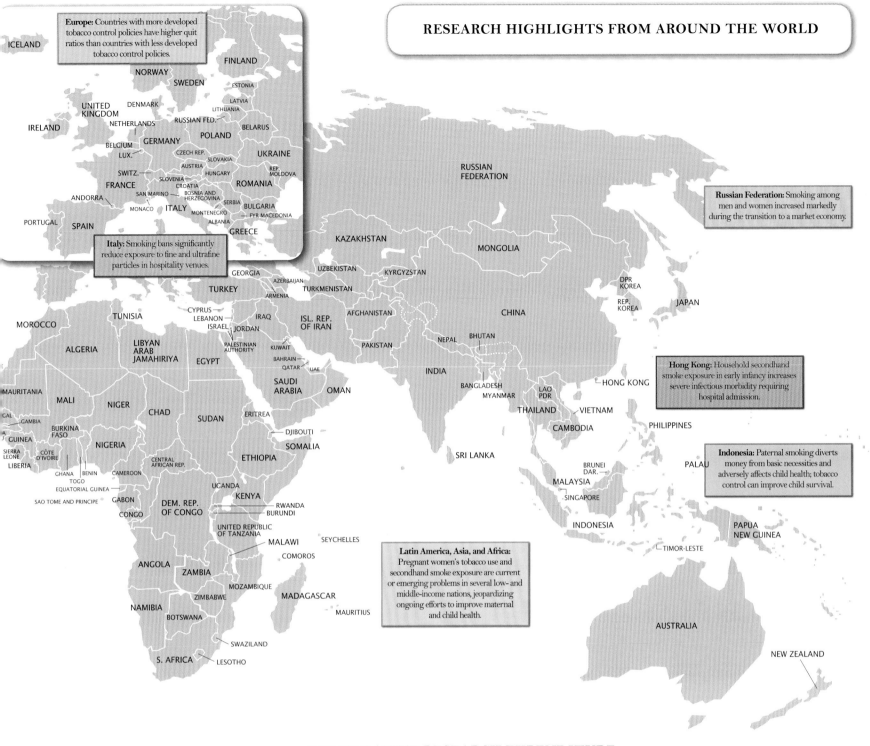

Europe: Countries with more developed tobacco control policies have higher quit ratios than countries with less developed tobacco control policies.

Italy: Smoking bans significantly reduce exposure to fine and ultrafine particles in hospitality venues.

Russian Federation: Smoking among men and women increased markedly during the transition to a market economy.

Hong Kong: Household secondhand smoke exposure in early infancy increases severe infectious morbidity requiring hospital admission.

Indonesia: Paternal smoking diverts money from basic necessities and adversely affects child health; tobacco control can improve child survival.

Latin America, Asia, and Africa: Pregnant women's tobacco use and secondhand smoke exposure are current or emerging problems in several low- and middle-income nations, jeopardizing ongoing efforts to improve maternal and child health.

COMPARATIVE RESEARCH EXPENDITURE

U.S. National Institutes of Health spending on research funding for major health problems, 2007, US$ per related death

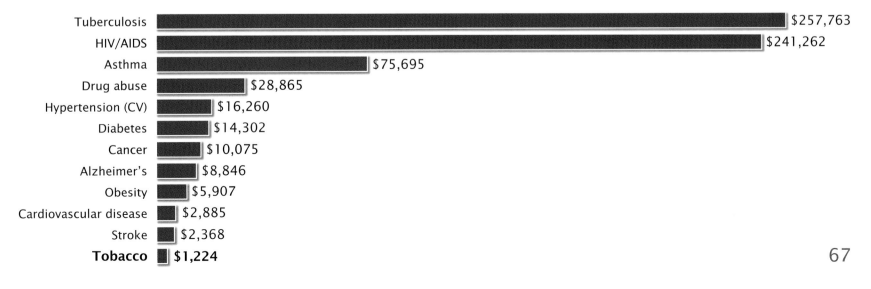

Tuberculosis	$257,763
HIV/AIDS	$241,262
Asthma	$75,695
Drug abuse	$28,865
Hypertension (CV)	$16,260
Diabetes	$14,302
Cancer	$10,075
Alzheimer's	$8,846
Obesity	$5,907
Cardiovascular disease	$2,885
Stroke	$2,368
Tobacco	$1,224

CHAPTER 21

CAPACITY BUILDING

"To see what is right, and not to do it, is want of courage or of principle."
—CONFUCIUS (551–479 BCE)

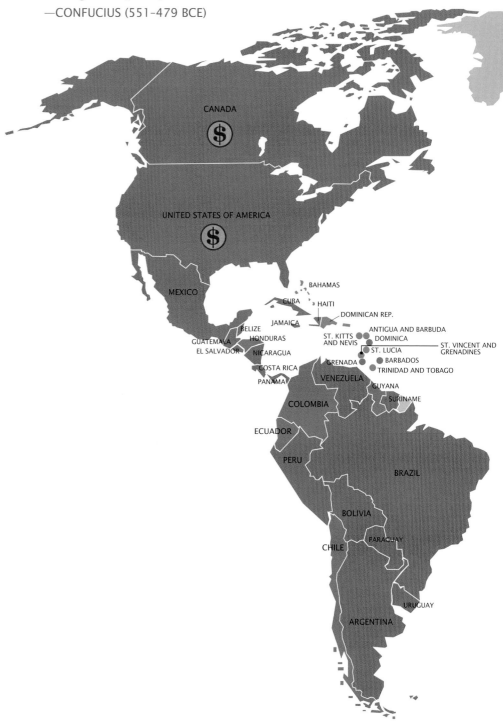

Tobacco control capacity refers to a nation's ability to achieve individual, institutional, and societal goals for reducing tobacco consumption. Many countries lack the capacity to counter the tobacco industry's incursions or to fully implement the articles of the Framework Convention on Tobacco Control (FCTC). Building national capacity for tobacco control entails leadership development, policy advocacy, investment in surveillance infrastructure, and consistent enforcement of tobacco control laws.

Fostering strong and effective non-governmental organizations and institutions is crucial to national capacity building. Organizations can empower citizens with information, skills, and resources to control tobacco and promote public health.

The World Health Organization, Bloomberg Initiative to Reduce Tobacco Use, the Bill & Melinda Gates Foundation, the Framework Convention Alliance, and GLOBALink have

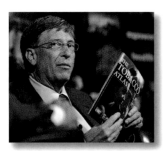

made enormous contributions to building national tobacco control capacity. As of July 2008, the Bloomberg Philanthropies have funded 73 projects in 31 countries. Philanthropists Michael Bloomberg and Bill and Melinda Gates's commitment (to date) of $500 million over seven years (2006–2013) more than triples the available resources to control tobacco in low- and middle-resource countries.

Financial resources help to level the playing field against multibillion-dollar tobacco companies, but even at low resource levels, each nation, institution, and individual has the capacity to adopt policies and practices that reduce and eliminate the scourge of tobacco.

A SELECTION OF ORGANIZATIONS FUNDING GLOBAL TOBACCO CONTROL

- American Cancer Society
- Bill & Melinda Gates Foundation
- Bloomberg Philanthropies
- Cancer Council Australia
- Cancer Research UK
- Framework Convention Alliance
- French Cancer League
- Global Tobacco Research Network
- International Union for Health Promotion and Education
- Norwegian Cancer Society
- Open Society Institute
- Program for Appropriate Technology in Health (PATH Canada)
- Romania Tobacco Control
- Swedish International Development Agency
- World Health Organization Tobacco Free Initiative (WHO TFI)
- World Lung Foundation

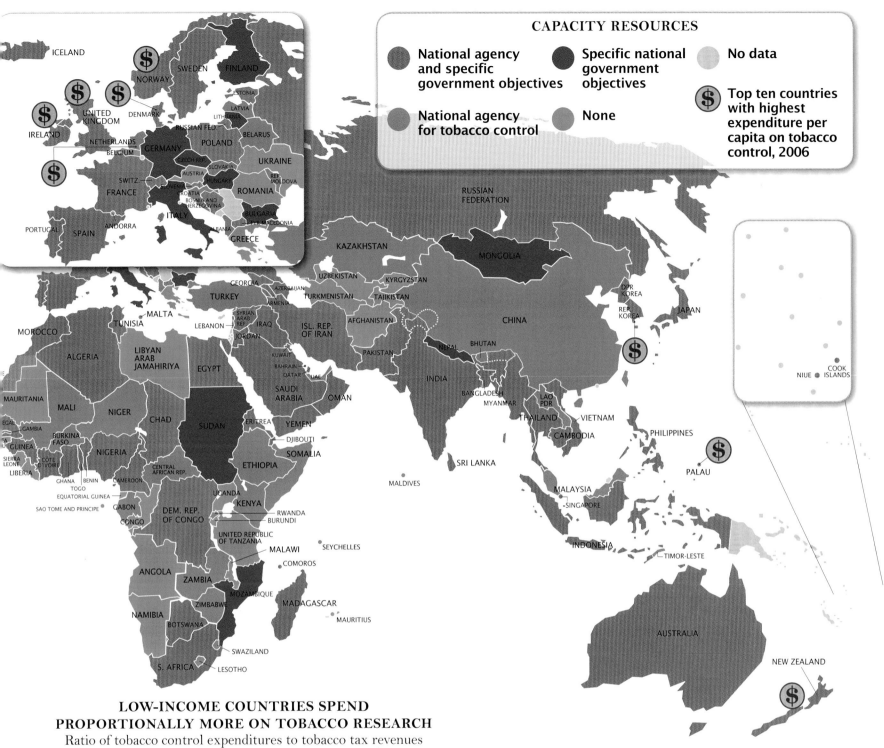

CAPACITY RESOURCES

- National agency and specific government objectives
- National agency for tobacco control
- Specific national government objectives
- None
- No data
- $ Top ten countries with highest expenditure per capita on tobacco control, 2006

LOW-INCOME COUNTRIES SPEND PROPORTIONALLY MORE ON TOBACCO RESEARCH

Ratio of tobacco control expenditures to tobacco tax revenues

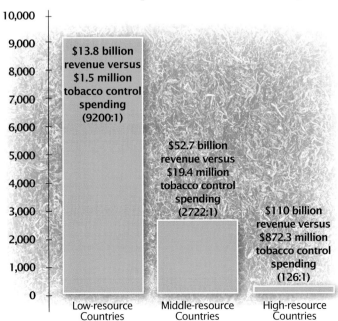

$13.8 billion revenue versus $1.5 million tobacco control spending (9200:1)

$52.7 billion revenue versus $19.4 million tobacco control spending (2722:1)

$110 billion revenue versus $872.3 million tobacco control spending (126:1)

Low-resource Countries

Middle-resource Countries

High-resource Countries

A higher ratio reflects weaker commitment to tobacco control.

"WE HAVE SEEN . . . the power of information to change the world, and right now, in villages and cities across the globe, the public health community is exposing the destructiveness of tobacco. . . ."

—Michael R. Bloomberg, 2008
Mayor of the City of New York

"THE CURE FOR this devastating epidemic is dependent not on medicines or vaccines, but on the concerted actions of government and civil society."

—Margaret Chan, 2008
Director General,
World Health Organization

69

WHO FRAMEWORK CONVENTION ON TOBACCO CONTROL

Salus populi suprema lex esto. (Let the welfare of the people be the supreme law.)
—CICERO (106-43 BCE)

The FCTC came into effect on February 27, 2005, and to date 162 of 192 World Health Organization member states have become parties to the Convention, making it one of the most rapidly embraced international treaties of all time. The Conference of Parties' secretariat has been established and meets annually to develop protocols and guidelines for implementation.

The treaty helps legislators realize that the tide of tobacco control is global and inevitable, good for both the wealth and health of nations. Not surprisingly, the tobacco industry was against a strong, legally binding FCTC, and sought voluntary agreements and self-regulating market mechanisms, which are essentially ineffective.

The tobacco industry need not fear the FCTC, as between 2010 and 2025 the number of smokers worldwide is predicted to rise from 1.4 billion to 1.7 billion, due mainly to population increases, even as smoking prevalence rates decline. Health economists predict that the FCTC will not harm national economies, even of tobacco-growing nations, because the FCTC deals primarily with demand reduction strategies, except for the control of smuggling. The treaty has mobilized resources, rallied hundreds of non-governmental organizations (NGO), encouraged government action, led to the political maturation of health ministries, and raised tobacco control awareness in other government ministries and departments.

The first protocol will be on illicit trade, and guidelines have been adopted to protect public health policies from the interference of the tobacco industry (Article 5.3); to ensure that truth about tobacco use be properly reflected in packaging and labeling of tobacco products, using picture-health warnings (Article 11); and to ban advertising, promotion, and sponsorship of tobacco products nationally and across borders (Article 13).

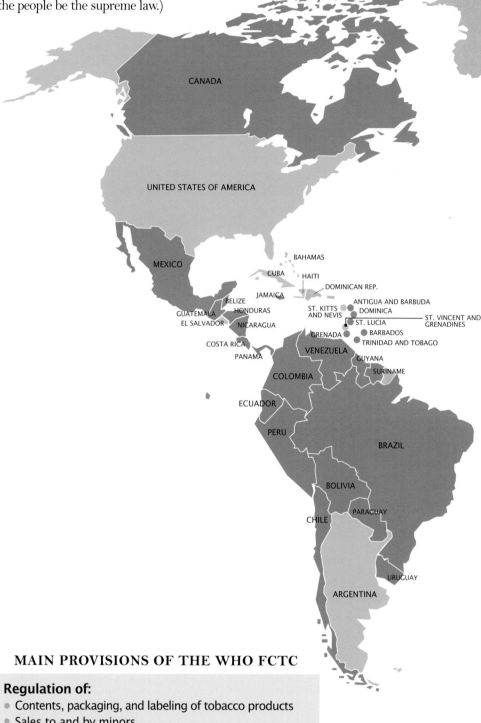

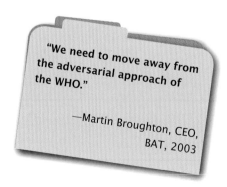

"We need to move away from the adversarial approach of the WHO."

—Martin Broughton, CEO, BAT, 2003

MAIN PROVISIONS OF THE WHO FCTC

Regulation of:
- Contents, packaging, and labeling of tobacco products
- Sales to and by minors
- Illicit trade in tobacco products
- Smoking at work and public places

Reduction in consumer demand by:
- Price and tax measures
- Comprehensive ban on tobacco advertising, promotion, and sponsorship
- Education, training, raising public awareness, and assistance with quitting

Protection of the environment and health of tobacco workers:
- Support for economically viable alternative activities
- Research, surveillance, and exchange of information
- Support for legislative action to deal with liability

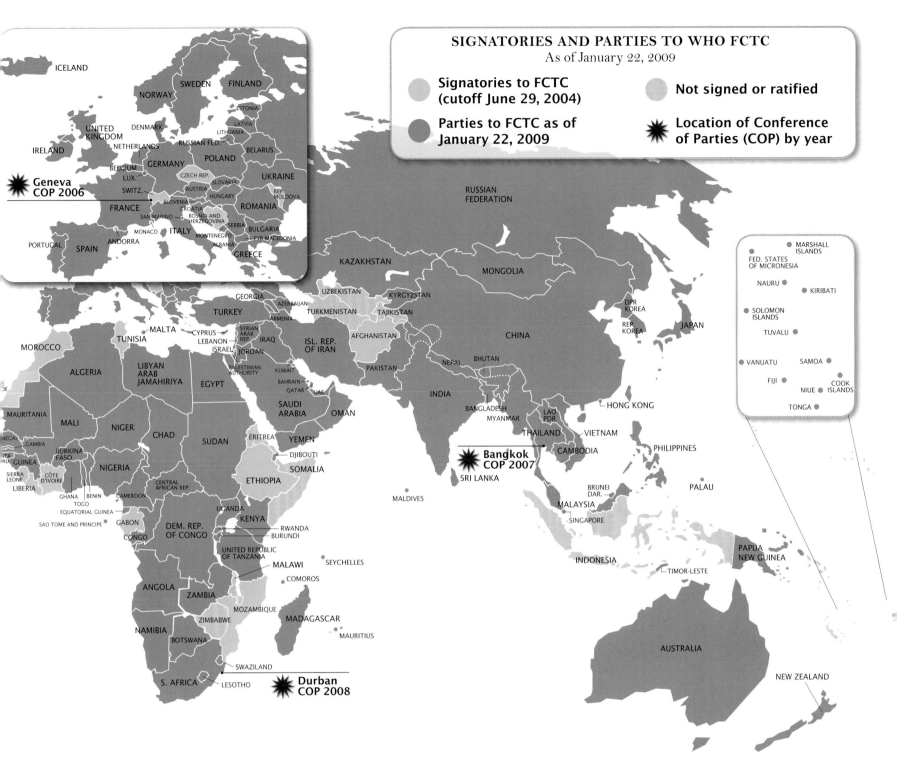

SIGNATORIES AND PARTIES TO WHO FCTC
As of January 22, 2009

- Signatories to FCTC (cutoff June 29, 2004)
- Parties to FCTC as of January 22, 2009
- Not signed or ratified
- ✸ Location of Conference of Parties (COP) by year

✸ Geneva COP 2006

✸ Bangkok COP 2007

✸ Durban COP 2008

WHAT WILL THE TOBACCO INDUSTRY DO?
Propagate the myth that the FCTC will harm the economy

Article 8 — Smoke-free areas:
- Argue for voluntary agreements
- Argue that smoke-free areas will harm the restaurant business
- Promote so-called accommodation policies
- Argue that smoke-free public places will lead to more smoking in the home

Article 13 — Bans on promotion:
- Seek to portray advertising as a consumer choice
- Argue advertising has no influence on demand, only consumer preference
- Exaggerate economic impact on advertisers, media, etc.
- Frame argument around "freedom of speech"
- Promote voluntary restrictions
- Seek partial restrictions
- Employ sophisticated strategies to circumvent laws

INITIAL TREATY PROTOCOLS AND GUIDELINES
(under negotiation)

Article	Topic	
15	Illicit trade	1st Protocol
5.3	Protection of public health policies from tobacco industry interference	Guideline
8	Protection from exposure to tobacco smoke	Guideline
9	Regulation of the contents of tobacco products	Guideline
10	Regulation of tobacco product disclosures	Guideline
11	Packaging and labeling of tobacco products	Guideline
12	Education, communication, training, and public awareness	Guideline
13	Tobacco advertising, promotion, and sponsorship	Guideline
14	Demand reduction measures concerning tobacco dependence and cessation	Guideline
26	Financial resources and assistance to developing countries and countries with economies in transition	Under discussion

CHAPTER 23

SMOKE-FREE AREAS

"Fears in the hospitality industry that smoking bans may damage business interests are largely unfounded."

—WORLD BANK, 2002

Smoking bans benefit nonsmokers and smokers alike. Nonsmokers are exposed to significantly less secondhand smoke, while smokers tend to smoke less, have greater cessation success, and have increased confidence in their ability to quit. These effects are greater under a comprehensive ban than under a partial one. When indoor smoking areas are allowed, ventilation is inadequate to eliminate secondhand smoke, and the reduction in smoking among smokers is less significant.

Smoking bans, relatively inexpensive to implement, produce immediate economic benefits to employers in the form of reduced accidental fire risk, lower insurance premiums, and less employee absenteeism.

Support is high for smoking bans in public places. In many countries with few regulations on smoke-free areas, the public is overwhelmingly in favor of establishing clean indoor air laws. In regions where smoking bans have been mandated by law, employees, customers, and business owners report high compliance and satisfaction with the results.

There is no safe level of exposure to secondhand smoke/environmental tobacco smoke. Attempts to control the toxic and carcinogenic properties of secondhand smoke by ventilation are futile, requiring tornado-strength rates of air flow. Among nonsmoking adults living in countries with extensive smoke-free law coverage, 12.5 percent were exposed to secondhand smoke, compared with 35.1 percent with limited coverage, and 45.9 percent with no law, and only 5 percent of the world's population is covered by comprehensive smoke-free laws.

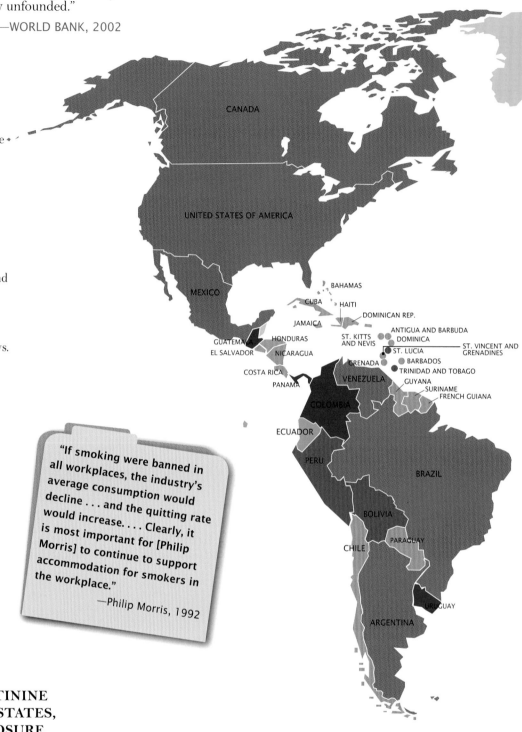

"If smoking were banned in all workplaces, the industry's average consumption would decline . . . and the quitting rate would increase. . . . Clearly, it is most important for [Philip Morris] to continue to support accommodation for smokers in the workplace."

—Philip Morris, 1992

DECREASE IN MEDIAN SERUM COTININE LEVELS IN NONSMOKERS, UNITED STATES, FOLLOWING REDUCTION IN EXPOSURE TO SECONDHAND SMOKE

Decrease between 1988–1991 and 1999–2002

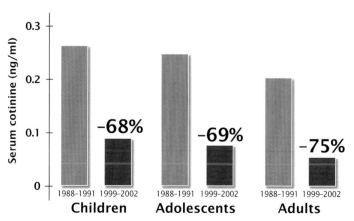

Serum cotinine (ng/ml)

-68% Children
-69% Adolescents
-75% Adults

1988-1991 1999-2002

UNITED STATES, 2007: Nonsmoking employees left unprotected from workplace secondhand smoke exposure had elevated levels of a tobacco-specific carcinogen in their bodies.

IRELAND, 2004: With smoke-free legislation, bar workers' exposure to secondhand smoke plunged from thirty hours per week to zero.

CHINA, 2007: Ninety percent of those living in large cities support a ban on smoking in public transport, schools, and hospitals. Eighty percent support a ban in the workplace.

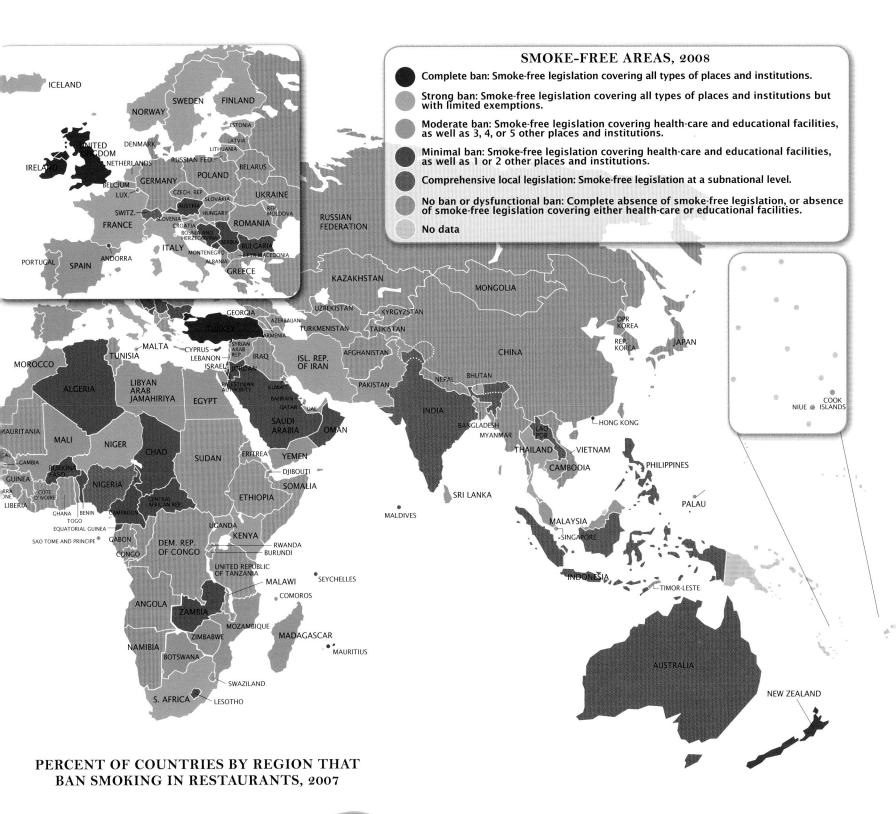

SMOKE-FREE AREAS, 2008

Complete ban: Smoke-free legislation covering all types of places and institutions.

Strong ban: Smoke-free legislation covering all types of places and institutions but with limited exemptions.

Moderate ban: Smoke-free legislation covering health-care and educational facilities, as well as 3, 4, or 5 other places and institutions.

Minimal ban: Smoke-free legislation covering health-care and educational facilities, as well as 1 or 2 other places and institutions.

Comprehensive local legislation: Smoke-free legislation at a subnational level.

No ban or dysfunctional ban: Complete absence of smoke-free legislation, or absence of smoke-free legislation covering either health-care or educational facilities.

No data

PERCENT OF COUNTRIES BY REGION THAT BAN SMOKING IN RESTAURANTS, 2007

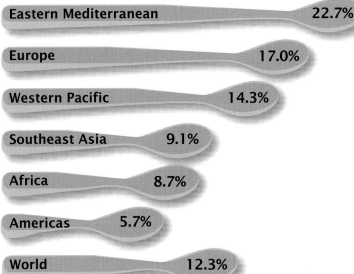

Eastern Mediterranean — 22.7%
Europe — 17.0%
Western Pacific — 14.3%
Southeast Asia — 9.1%
Africa — 8.7%
Americas — 5.7%
World — 12.3%

NO LOSS OF RESTAURANT AND BAR SALES AFTER SMOKE-FREE INITIATIVE
California, USA, 1992–2006

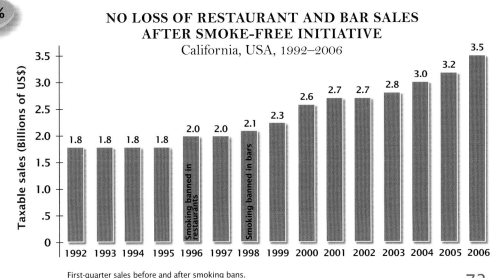

Taxable sales (Billions of US$)

1992	1993	1994	1995	1996	1997	1998	1999	2000	2001	2002	2003	2004	2005	2006
1.8	1.8	1.8	1.8	2.0	2.0	2.1	2.3	2.6	2.7	2.7	2.8	3.0	3.2	3.5

Smoking banned in restaurants

Smoking banned in bars

First-quarter sales before and after smoking bans.

MARKETING BANS

"Bans on advertising and promotion prove effective, but only if they are comprehensive, covering all media and all uses of brand names and logos. . . . If governments only ban tobacco advertising in one or two [types of] media, the industry will simply shift its advertising expenditures, with no effect on overall consumption."

—HENRY SAFFER, NATIONAL BUREAU OF ECONOMIC RESEARCH, USA, 2000

Tobacco marketing increases cigarette consumption and seduces new smokers into addiction, negating public health efforts to control tobacco. Recognizing this, many countries have imposed some restrictions on tobacco marketing. However, partial restrictions are ineffective in reducing smoking because tobacco companies redirect their marketing efforts to available venues. Voluntary agreements are also inadequate because they are unenforceable.

In the face of broadening advertising bans, tobacco companies have become ever more creative in their attempts to lure new consumers into addiction. Brand stretching, event promotion, retailer incentives, sponsorship and advertising through international media, cross-border advertising, and promotional packaging are some of the ways that the tobacco industry circumvents advertising bans.

Only comprehensive official bans on all forms of tobacco advertising, marketing, sponsorship, and promotion are effective at reducing population smoking rates.

Parents also can do their part at the individual level by protecting children from exposure to depictions of smoking in movies. Parental restrictions and parental nonsmoking strongly predict lower risk of smoking initiation among youth.

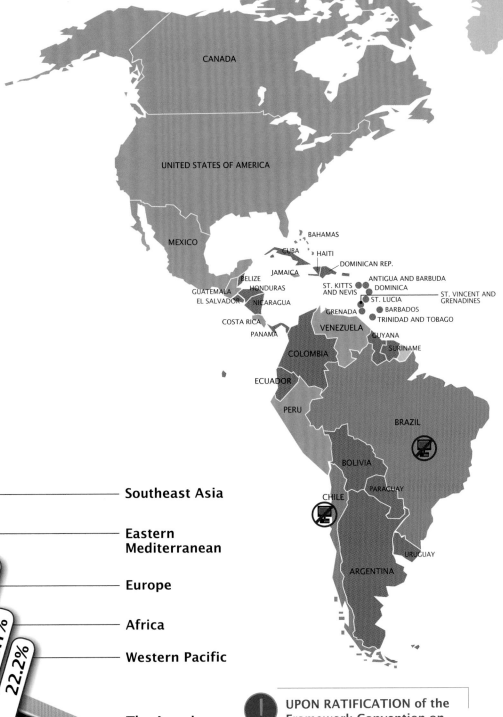

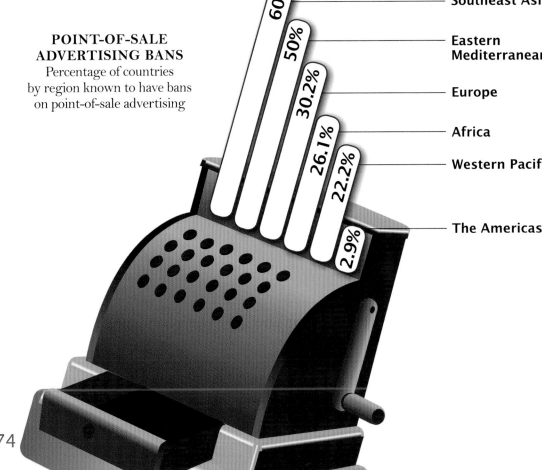

POINT-OF-SALE ADVERTISING BANS
Percentage of countries by region known to have bans on point-of-sale advertising

- 60% — Southeast Asia
- 50% — Eastern Mediterranean
- 30.2% — Europe
- 26.1% — Africa
- 22.2% — Western Pacific
- 2.9% — The Americas

UPON RATIFICATION of the Framework Convention on Tobacco Control (FCTC), countries must implement a comprehensive advertising ban within five years.

COMPREHENSIVE advertising bans can reduce smoking rates by 6 percent per year.

ADVERTISING BANS may be even more effective in low- and middle-resource countries than in high-resource countries.

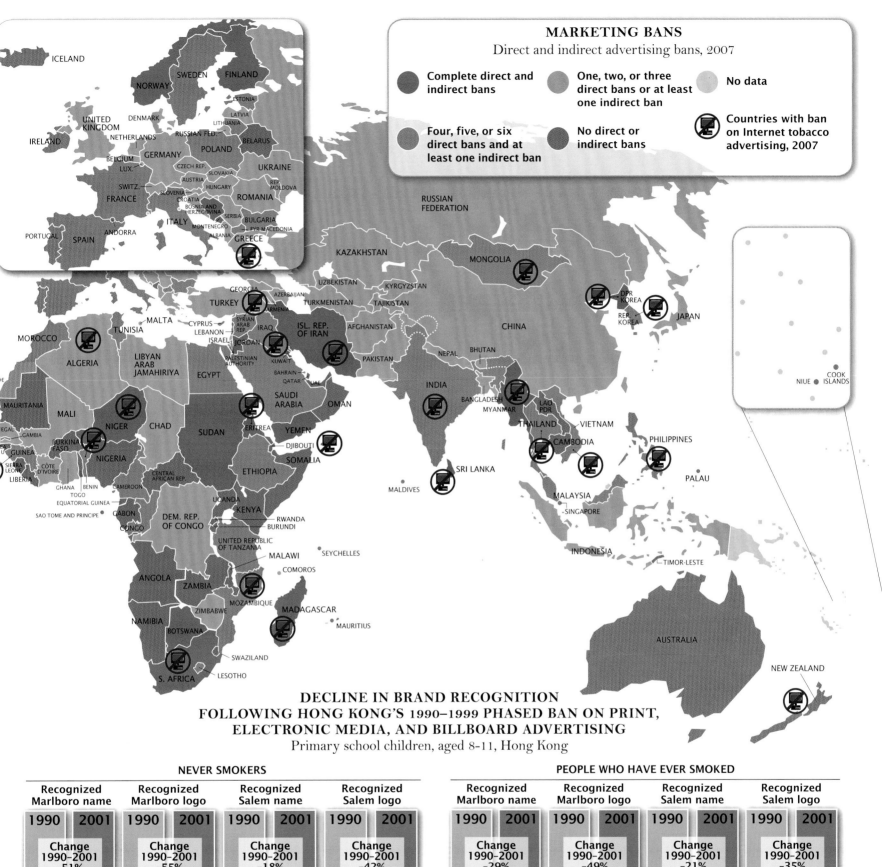

MARKETING BANS
Direct and indirect advertising bans, 2007

- Complete direct and indirect bans
- One, two, or three direct bans or at least one indirect ban
- No data
- Four, five, or six direct bans and at least one indirect ban
- No direct or indirect bans
- Countries with ban on Internet tobacco advertising, 2007

DECLINE IN BRAND RECOGNITION
FOLLOWING HONG KONG'S 1990–1999 PHASED BAN ON PRINT, ELECTRONIC MEDIA, AND BILLBOARD ADVERTISING
Primary school children, aged 8-11, Hong Kong

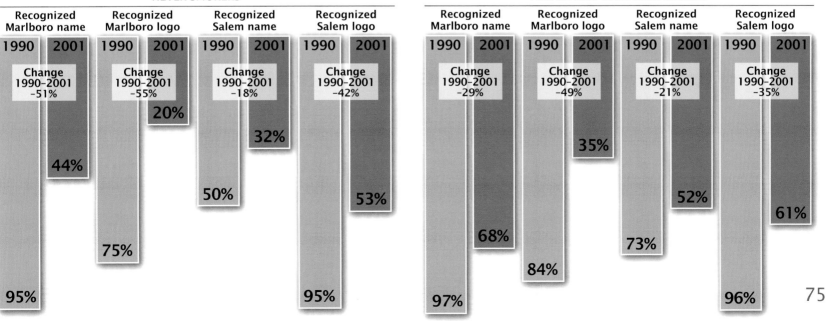

NEVER SMOKERS				PEOPLE WHO HAVE EVER SMOKED			
Recognized Marlboro name	Recognized Marlboro logo	Recognized Salem name	Recognized Salem logo	Recognized Marlboro name	Recognized Marlboro logo	Recognized Salem name	Recognized Salem logo
1990 / 2001	1990 / 2001	1990 / 2001	1990 / 2001	1990 / 2001	1990 / 2001	1990 / 2001	1990 / 2001
Change 1990-2001 -51%	Change 1990-2001 -55%	Change 1990-2001 -18%	Change 1990-2001 -42%	Change 1990-2001 -29%	Change 1990-2001 -49%	Change 1990-2001 -21%	Change 1990-2001 -35%
44%	20%	32%	53%	68%	35%	52%	61%
95%	75%	50%	95%	97%	84%	73%	96%

75

PRODUCT LABELING

"Size does matter."
—DAVID SIMPSON, ON HEALTH WARNINGS, 2004

Health warnings on the packaging of all tobacco products are guaranteed to reach all users. Since the 1960s, warning labels on cigarette packs have been used as a way to communicate risks associated with smoking and encouragement to quit. Health warnings on cigarette packs are now required in most countries of the world, and laws are steadily increasing the required size of the warning, strengthening the content, and enhancing the graphic design.

In one of its strongest provisions, Article 11 of the WHO Framework Convention on Tobacco Control (FCTC) compels signatories, within three years of ratification, to require tobacco product health warnings that cover at least 30 percent, and preferably 50 percent, of the visible area on a cigarette pack. Warnings should be extended to all forms of smoking and smokeless tobacco.

Efforts to correct decades of consumer misperceptions about light cigarettes must extend beyond simply removing "light" and "mild" brand descriptors.

Plain packaging, displaying only the brand name and the health warning with no use of color, logo, or promotional graphic design, increases both prominence and credibility of health warnings. Plain packaging requirements are consistent with restrictions on tobacco advertising because promotional packaging is one of the industry's most important advertising tools.

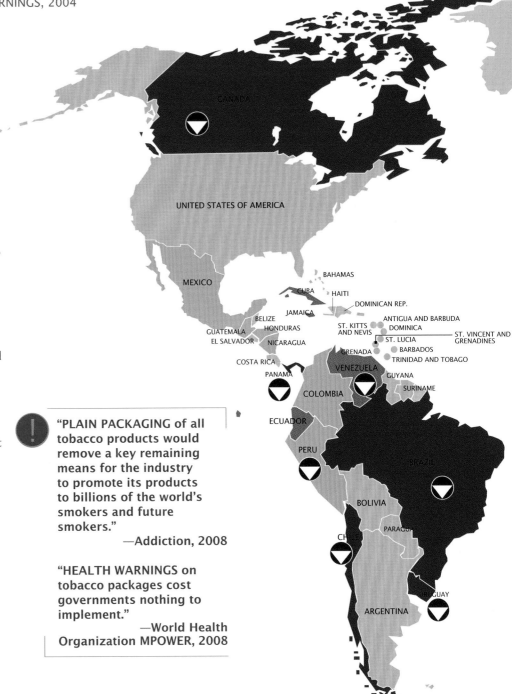

"PLAIN PACKAGING of all tobacco products would remove a key remaining means for the industry to promote its products to billions of the world's smokers and future smokers."
—Addiction, 2008

"HEALTH WARNINGS on tobacco packages cost governments nothing to implement."
—World Health Organization MPOWER, 2008

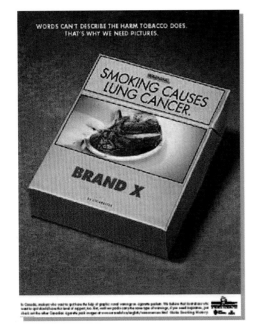

MISLEADING LIGHTS

Light/mild smokers who believe that "light" or "mild" cigarettes reduce the risks of smoking without having to give up smoking, Canada, 2003.

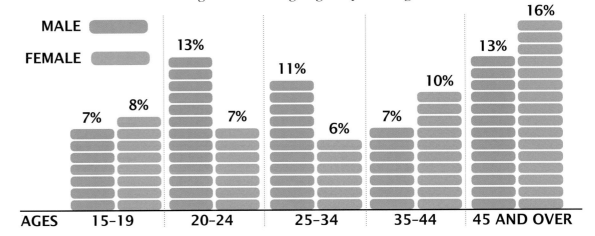

MALE

FEMALE

AGES	15-19	20-24	25-34	35-44	45 AND OVER
MALE	7%	13%	11%	7%	13%
FEMALE	8%	7%	6%	10%	16%

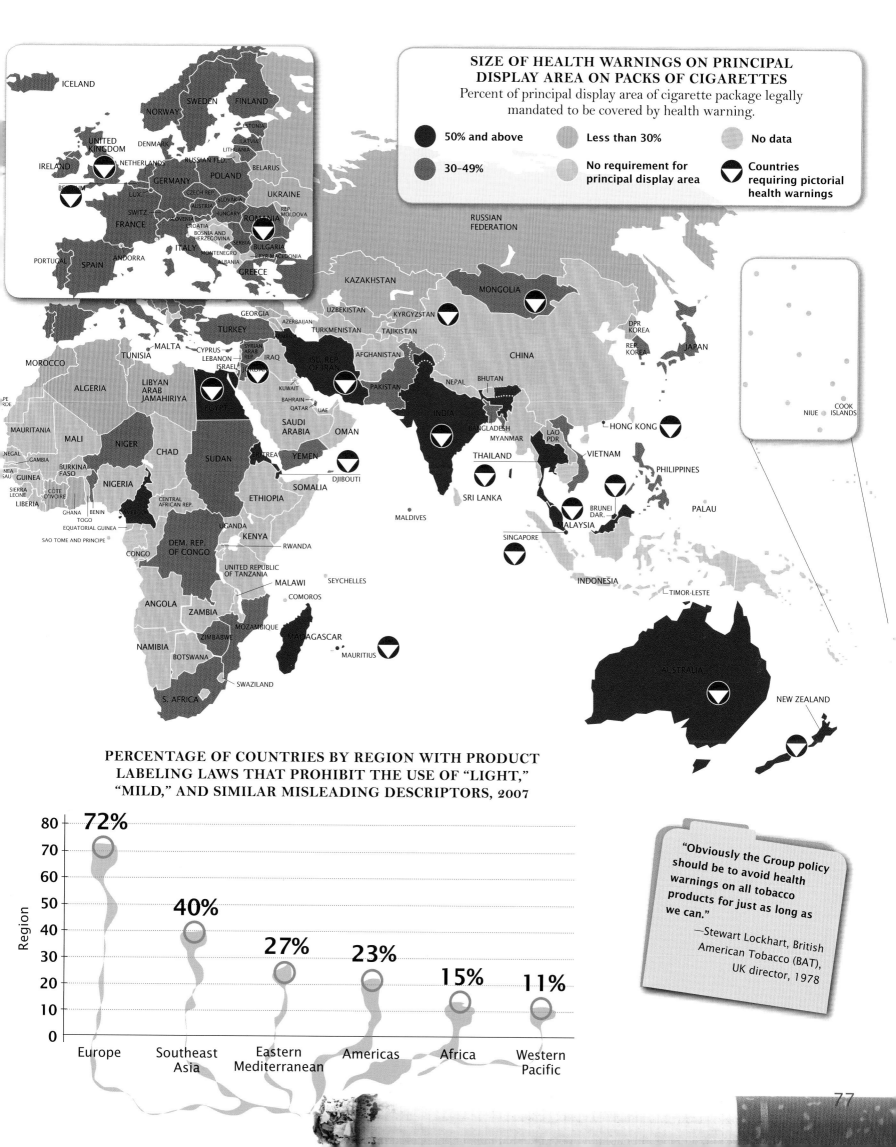

SIZE OF HEALTH WARNINGS ON PRINCIPAL DISPLAY AREA ON PACKS OF CIGARETTES

Percent of principal display area of cigarette package legally mandated to be covered by health warning.

- 50% and above
- 30–49%
- Less than 30%
- No requirement for principal display area
- No data
- Countries requiring pictorial health warnings

PERCENTAGE OF COUNTRIES BY REGION WITH PRODUCT LABELING LAWS THAT PROHIBIT THE USE OF "LIGHT," "MILD," AND SIMILAR MISLEADING DESCRIPTORS, 2007

Region

- Europe: 72%
- Southeast Asia: 40%
- Eastern Mediterranean: 27%
- Americas: 23%
- Africa: 15%
- Western Pacific: 11%

"Obviously the Group policy should be to avoid health warnings on all tobacco products for just as long as we can."

—Stewart Lockhart, British American Tobacco (BAT), UK director, 1978

PUBLIC HEALTH CAMPAIGNS

*"The irony is that the tobacco industry uses images of health to sell death,
while health organizations use images of death to sell health."*

—YUSSUF SALOOJEE, WORLD LUNG CONFERENCE, CAPETOWN, 2007

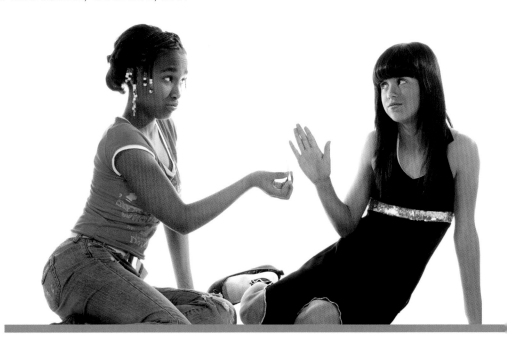

Legislative and tax interventions to reduce smoking rates alone are unlikely to be accepted without public awareness and support for tobacco control interventions. Mass communication, health education, and reliable information are essential elements for tobacco control success.

Most governments and school systems have meager budgets to develop, implement, and sustain comprehensive school-based programs, including sound policies, cessation services, and effective anti-tobacco curricula. In many countries, especially where health education is under-funded and under-resourced, the tobacco industry seizes the opportunity to burnish its public image by funding youth smoking prevention programs. Unsurprisingly, most industry-sponsored youth programs employ measures known to have minimal impact on youth smoking uptake. In many cases, they encourage smoking by associating the behavior with aspirational ideals of maturity and freedom (smoking as an "adult choice").

Much of the world's health education happens outside the classroom: through media, movies, popular culture, and the Internet. Earned media, such as unpaid news stories about tobacco control activities, and social media are important forms of tobacco control promotion. Because social networks are powerful propagators of smoking behavior, social networking Web sites are among the powerful new media platforms available for dialogue, support, and dissemination of anti-smoking health information.

 "NO SENSIBLE, ethical person will take money from drug dealers for a youth programme to prevent drug abuse. No one . . . would accept money from child pornographers to teach children about sexual harassment. So why should governments . . . accept money from the tobacco industry to teach young people not to smoke?"

—World Health Organization Western Pacific Regional Office, Tobacco Free Initiative, 2002

YOUTH PREVENTION PROGRAMS
Effective versus ineffective measures. Campaigns sponsored by the tobacco industry tend to be ineffective.

LIKELY TO BE EFFECTIVE *If framed within a comprehensive tobacco control program*	LIKELY TO BE INEFFECTIVE *Establishes youth prevention and education as stand-alone issues*
Does not position smoking and tobacco use as a "grown-up activity" but something that affects all ages	Positions tobacco as "adult" and forbidden. Advocates messages such as: • "Youth should not smoke." • "Smoking is an adult decision." • "Only adults should smoke." • "Obey the law." • "Just say no."
Supports tobacco tax increases	No mention of tobacco tax increases
Supports total advertising bans	Stresses peer pressure as the main cause of teen smoking, without acknowledging the role of advertising and promotion, especially those targeted at youth
Supports comprehensive smoke-free areas	Ignores the issue of smoke-free areas
Bans display of tobacco products (e.g., as in Thailand). Limiting the distribution channels (some store chains/pharmacies stopped selling tobacco)	Emphasizes restriction of access to tobacco products to youth through ID cards, signs prohibiting sales to minors, policies to raise the age limit for tobacco sales
Emphasizes that nicotine is addictive	Depicts smoking as an "adult choice"
Discusses risks associated with smoking to people of all ages	Depicts "youth smoking" as the only problem
Addresses cessation among all smokers, young and adult	Does not address cessation at any age
Shows how the tobacco industry targets young people	Campaigns funded by the tobacco industry

WHO World No Tobacco Day campaign themes

1988	Tobacco or Health: Choose Health
1989	Women and Tobacco
1990	Growing Up Without Tobacco
1991	Tobacco in Public Places and on Public Transport
1992	Tobacco at the Workplace
1993	Health Services, including Health Personnel, Against Tobacco
1994	The Media Against Tobacco
1995	The Economics of Tobacco
1996	Sports and the Arts Without Tobacco
1997	"United for a Tobacco-Free World"
1998	Growing Up Without Tobacco
1999	Cessation
2000	Tobacco Kills, Don't Be Duped
2001	Secondhand Smoke Kills. Let's Clear the Air
2002	Tobacco-Free Sports: Play It Clean
2003	Tobacco-Free Film/Tobacco-Free Fashion
2004	Tobacco and Poverty
2005	Health Professionals Against Tobacco
2006	Tobacco: Deadly in Any Form or Disguise
2007	Smoke-Free Environments
2008	Tobacco-Free Youth
2009	Tobacco Health Warnings

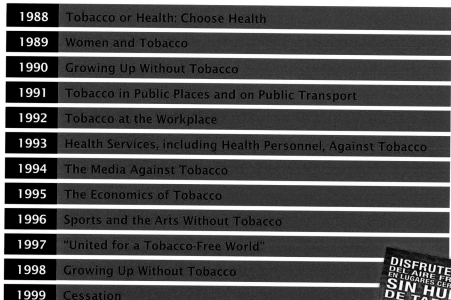

DISFRUTEMOS DEL AIRE FRESCO EN LUGARES CERRADOS SIN HUMO DE TABACO

Los niños que respiran el humo de tabaco padecen más enfermedades respiratorias como asma, bronquitis y neumonía.

Respirar aire sin humo de tabaco nos beneficia a todos.

PORQUE TODOS RESPIRAMOS LO MISMO

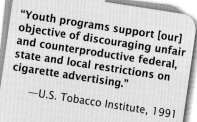

"Youth programs support [our] objective of discouraging unfair and counterproductive federal, state and local restrictions on cigarette advertising."
—U.S. Tobacco Institute, 1991

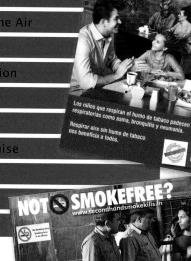

NOT SMOKEFREE?
www.secondhandsmokekills.in

FINE

National Tobacco Control Program
Government of India.

SMOKEFREE   COSTS   BENEFITS   COTPA   SIGNAGE   RESOURCES   CONTACT US

COTPA SIGNAGE
Signage Specifications

COTPA Signage
Point Of Smoking (POS) Signage

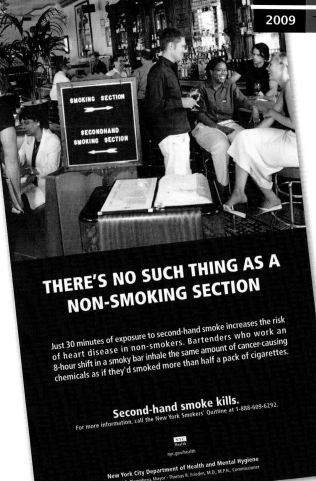

THERE'S NO SUCH THING AS A NON-SMOKING SECTION

SMOKING SECTION →

SECONDHAND SMOKING SECTION →

Just 30 minutes of exposure to second-hand smoke increases the risk of heart disease in non-smokers. Bartenders who work an 8-hour shift in a smoky bar inhale the same amount of cancer-causing chemicals as if they'd smoked more than half a pack of cigarettes.

Second-hand smoke kills.
For more information, call the New York Smokers' Quitline at 1-888-609-6292.

NYC Health
nyc.gov/health

New York City Department of Health and Mental Hygiene
Michael R. Bloomberg, Mayor · Thomas R. Frieden, M.D., M.P.H., Commissioner

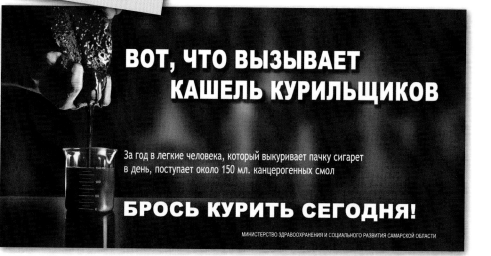

ВОТ, ЧТО ВЫЗЫВАЕТ КАШЕЛЬ КУРИЛЬЩИКОВ

За год в легкие человека, который выкуривает пачку сигарет в день, поступает около 150 мл. канцерогенных смол

БРОСЬ КУРИТЬ СЕГОДНЯ!

МИНИСТЕРСТВО ЗДРАВООХРАНЕНИЯ И СОЦИАЛЬНОГО РАЗВИТИЯ САМАРСКОЙ ОБЛАСТИ

CHAPTER 27

QUITTING SMOKING

"[Ten years ago] all we had to offer was going cold turkey or nicotine gum. . . . The good news for smokers is that people now have a choice. There's never been a better time to quit."

—MICHAEL C. FIORE, CHAIRPERSON, SUBCOMMITTEE ON CESSATION, U.S. DEPARTMENT OF HEALTH AND HUMAN SERVICES INTERAGENCY COMMITTEE ON SMOKING AND HEALTH

Smoking's harm is immediately reduced and can be virtually eliminated over time after quitting, even for lifelong smokers. It is never too late to quit! Advanced tobacco control policies can help increase quit rates, a prerequisite for achieving significant reductions in smoking-related deaths during the first half of the 21st century.

Many people kick the habit easily while others struggle through a difficult cycle of addiction. Quitting is possible and is increasingly becoming the norm. Many countries now have more ex-smokers than current smokers.

Most ex-smokers quit successfully on their own ("cold turkey"), but an increasing number of programs and aids are available to help liberate smokers from their addiction. Nicotine replacement therapies (gum, patch, and inhaler) and pharmacologic agents, such as bupropion and varenicline, are available in many countries.

Communication technologies—such as telephone quitlines, text messaging, interactive telephony, and online counseling—offer important support. Psychological and behavioral therapies, including behavior modification, hypnosis, meditation, and acupuncture, also have been employed.

Cessation programs change individual lives, reshape social norms and community values, and foster a world where children are less likely to casually experiment with cigarettes and where adults gain confidence in their ability to quit.

Within hours of quitting, some of the damage done by smoking begins to reverse. By one year, the risk of coronary heart disease is decreased to half that of a smoker. After five to fifteen years, the risk of a stroke is reduced virtually to that of people who have never smoked. Cancer risk also reduces significantly over the decade after quitting.

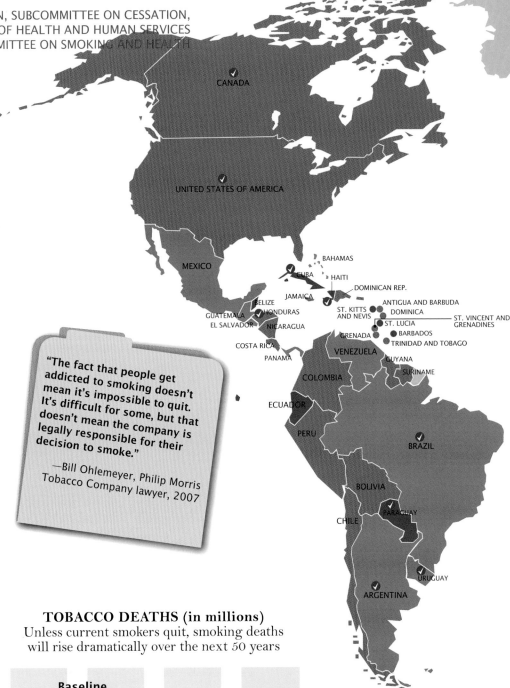

"The fact that people get addicted to smoking doesn't mean it's impossible to quit. It's difficult for some, but that doesn't mean the company is legally responsible for their decision to smoke."

—Bill Ohlemeyer, Philip Morris Tobacco Company lawyer, 2007

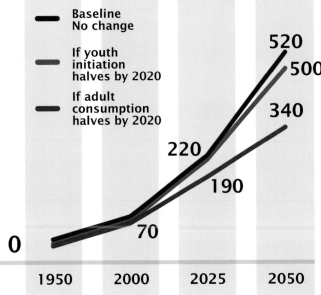

TOBACCO DEATHS (in millions)

Unless current smokers quit, smoking deaths will rise dramatically over the next 50 years

Baseline No change

If youth initiation halves by 2020

If adult consumption halves by 2020

520

500

340

220

190

70

0

1950 2000 2025 2050

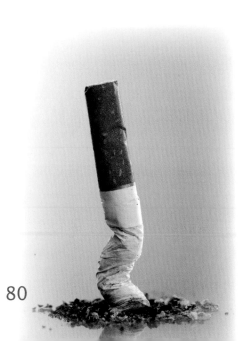

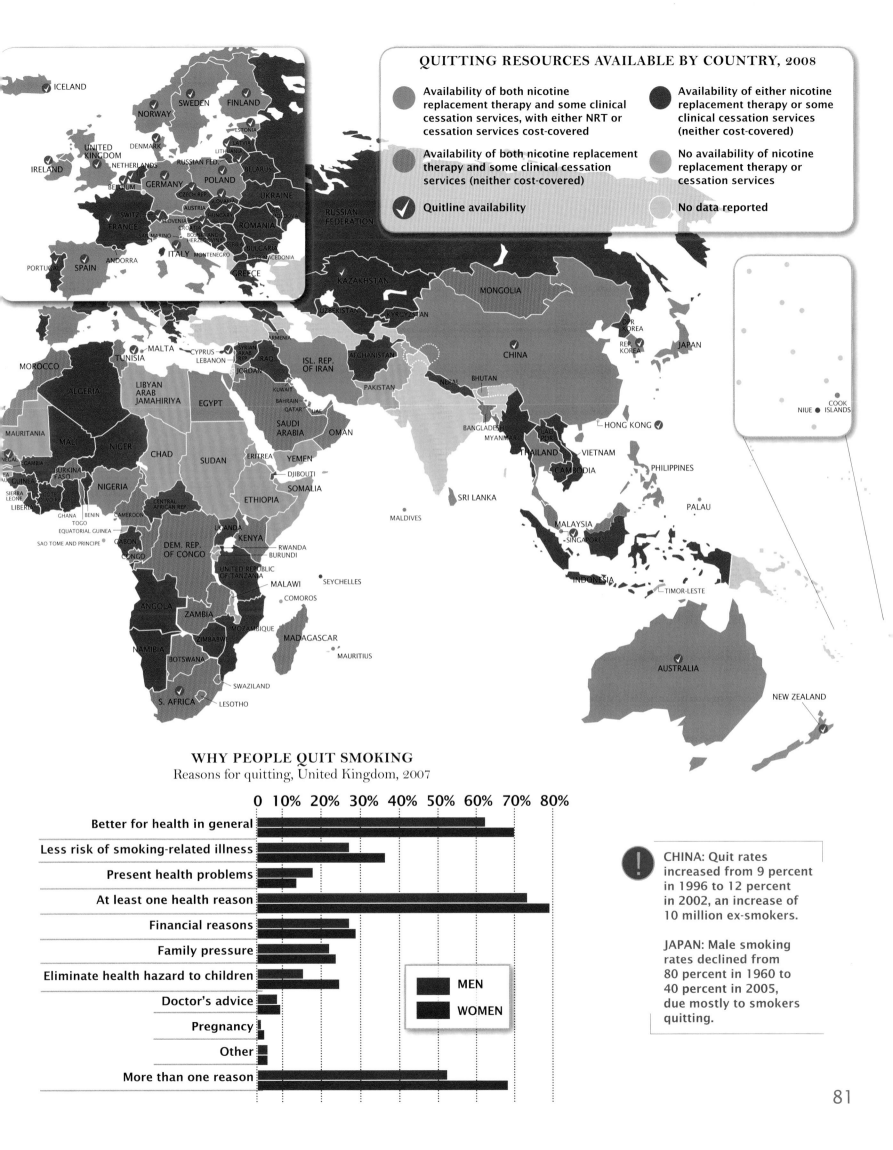

QUITTING RESOURCES AVAILABLE BY COUNTRY, 2008

- Availability of both nicotine replacement therapy and some clinical cessation services, with either NRT or cessation services cost-covered
- Availability of both nicotine replacement therapy and some clinical cessation services (neither cost-covered)
- ✓ Quitline availability
- Availability of either nicotine replacement therapy or some clinical cessation services (neither cost-covered)
- No availability of nicotine replacement therapy or cessation services
- No data reported

WHY PEOPLE QUIT SMOKING
Reasons for quitting, United Kingdom, 2007

0 10% 20% 30% 40% 50% 60% 70% 80%

- Better for health in general
- Less risk of smoking-related illness
- Present health problems
- At least one health reason
- Financial reasons
- Family pressure
- Eliminate health hazard to children
- Doctor's advice
- Pregnancy
- Other
- More than one reason

MEN
WOMEN

CHINA: Quit rates increased from 9 percent in 1996 to 12 percent in 2002, an increase of 10 million ex-smokers.

JAPAN: Male smoking rates declined from 80 percent in 1960 to 40 percent in 2005, due mostly to smokers quitting.

81

TOBACCO PRICES AND TAXES

"The Parties recognize that price and tax measures are an effective and important means of reducing tobacco consumption by various segments of the population."

—ARTICLE 6, FRAMEWORK CONVENTION ON TOBACCO CONTROL

Higher tobacco taxes that lead to higher cigarette prices encourage smokers to quit, reduce the number of cigarettes smoked, and prevent initiation among potential new users. A 10 percent increase in cigarette prices reduces cigarette demand by 2.5 to 5 percent. Youth, minorities, and low-income smokers are two to three times more likely than other smokers to quit or smoke less in response to price increases. Because cigarette prices strongly influence smoking initiation in youth, price increases significantly reduce long-term trends in cigarette consumption.

Tobacco tax increases are simple and effective tobacco control tools. In addition to reducing cigarette consumption, tobacco taxes typically generate higher tax revenues. These funds can be used to implement and enforce tobacco control policies and pay for related public health and social programs. This is good news for policy makers seeking to protect public health but wary about losing an important source of government revenue.

The World Health Organization's Framework Convention on Tobacco Control compels signatories to adopt tax and price policies that reduce tobacco consumption. The World Bank recommends that cigarette taxes (including value-added or sales taxes) account for two-thirds to four-fifths of the retail price of a pack of cigarettes. Cigarette tax increases significantly reduce cigarette consumption, improving both public health and national economic health.

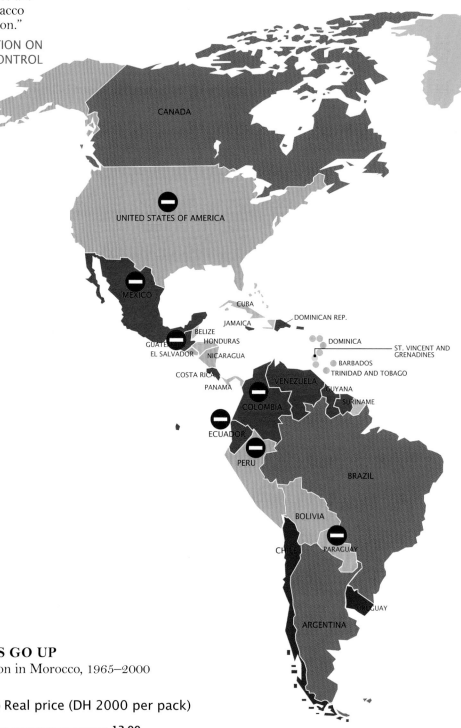

SMOKING GOES DOWN AS PRICES GO UP

Inflation-adjusted cigarette prices and cigarette consumption in Morocco, 1965–2000

Packs per adult year ⬤   ⬤ Real price (DH 2000 per pack)

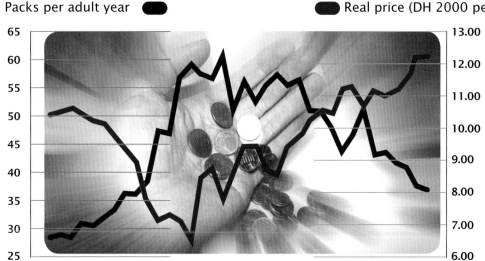

"With regard to taxation, it is clear that in the US, and in most countries in which we operate, tax is becoming a major threat to our existence."

—Philip Morris, 1985

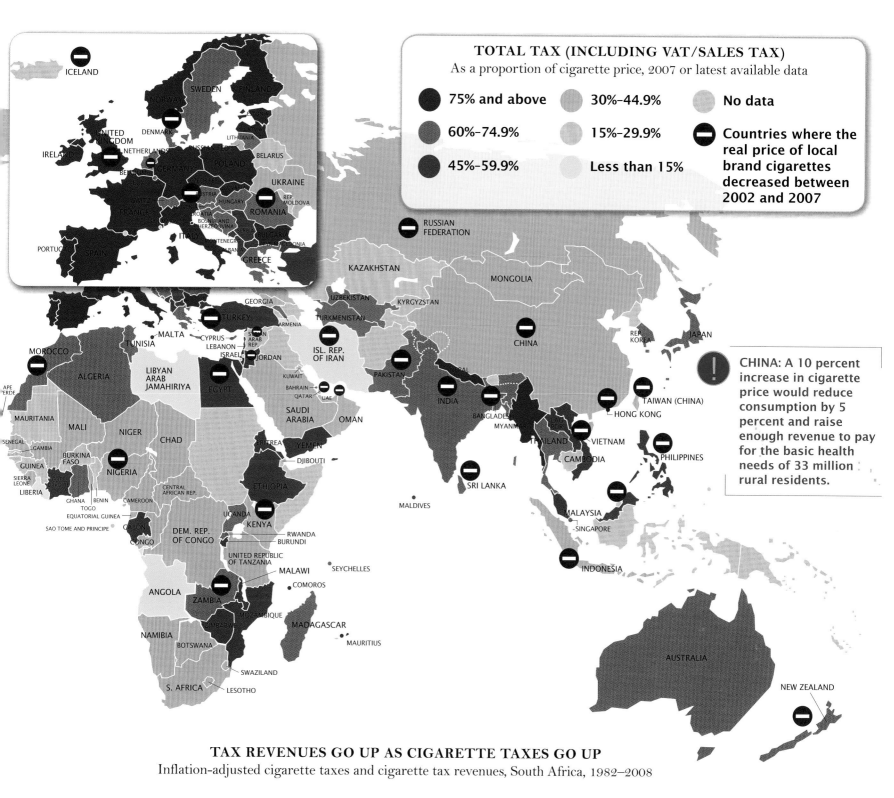

TOTAL TAX (INCLUDING VAT/SALES TAX)
As a proportion of cigarette price, 2007 or latest available data

- 75% and above
- 60%–74.9%
- 45%–59.9%
- 30%–44.9%
- 15%–29.9%
- Less than 15%
- No data
- Countries where the real price of local brand cigarettes decreased between 2002 and 2007

CHINA: A 10 percent increase in cigarette price would reduce consumption by 5 percent and raise enough revenue to pay for the basic health needs of 33 million rural residents.

TAX REVENUES GO UP AS CIGARETTE TAXES GO UP
Inflation-adjusted cigarette taxes and cigarette tax revenues, South Africa, 1982–2008

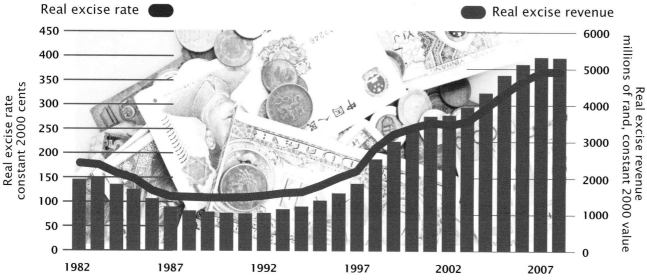

Real excise rate

Real excise revenue

CHAPTER 29

LITIGATION

"In order to protect themselves from smoking and health-related claims in litigation . . . they suppressed, concealed, and terminated scientific research; they destroyed documents including scientific reports and studies; and they repeatedly and intentionally improperly asserted the attorney-client and work product privileges over many thousands of documents (not just pages) to thwart disclosure . . . and to shield those documents from the harsh light of day."

—JUDGE GLADYS KESSLER,
U.S. DISTRICT COURT, 2006

The modern era of tobacco litigation began with a personal injury lawsuit in the United States in 1954. For more than 40 years, the tobacco industry boasted it had not lost a single case, but this has changed. A seminal judgment in 1994 released into the public domain millions of pages of internal tobacco industry documents. These internal documents reveal that tobacco companies actively concealed their knowledge about the harmfulness of smoking and intentionally deceived governments, the media, and their clients—smokers—about the extent of death and disease caused by their products.

Litigation puts the industry on the political defensive, forces tobacco companies to the bargaining table, and results in large settlements, with the industry paying U.S. states billions of dollars per year. A landmark case was decided on August 17, 2006, when U.S. District Court Judge Gladys Kessler ruled that tobacco company defendants violated the Racketeer Influenced Corrupt Organizations (RICO) Act.

Lawsuits against the tobacco industry were spearheaded in the U.S. judicial system, but tobacco litigation is clearly increasing around the world. The World Health Organization encourages litigation for the purpose of tobacco control, advocating that individuals and governments consider taking legal action, where necessary, to address criminal activity, product liability, health-care cost recovery, and other civil torts. Increasing numbers and types of lawsuits are being pressed against tobacco companies in Brazil, Canada, Israel, Italy, Nigeria, Poland, Turkey, and elsewhere.

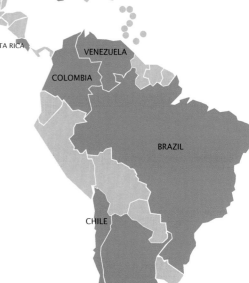

A RANGE OF LAWSUITS

Types of cases pending against Philip Morris, Philip Morris International, and affiliates (as of February 2008, U.S.)

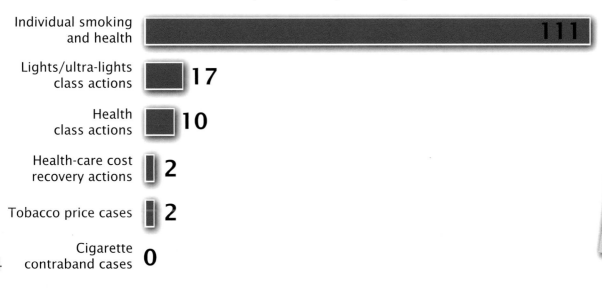

Individual smoking and health	111
Lights/ultra-lights class actions	17
Health class actions	10
Health-care cost recovery actions	2
Tobacco price cases	2
Cigarette contraband cases	0

"There is also a risk that, regardless of the outcome of the litigation, negative publicity from the litigation and other factors might make smoking less acceptable to the public, enhance public restrictions on smoking, induce many similar lawsuits against JT and its subsidiaries, forcing them to deal with and bear the costs of such lawsuits, and so on."

—Japan Tobacco Inc., 2007

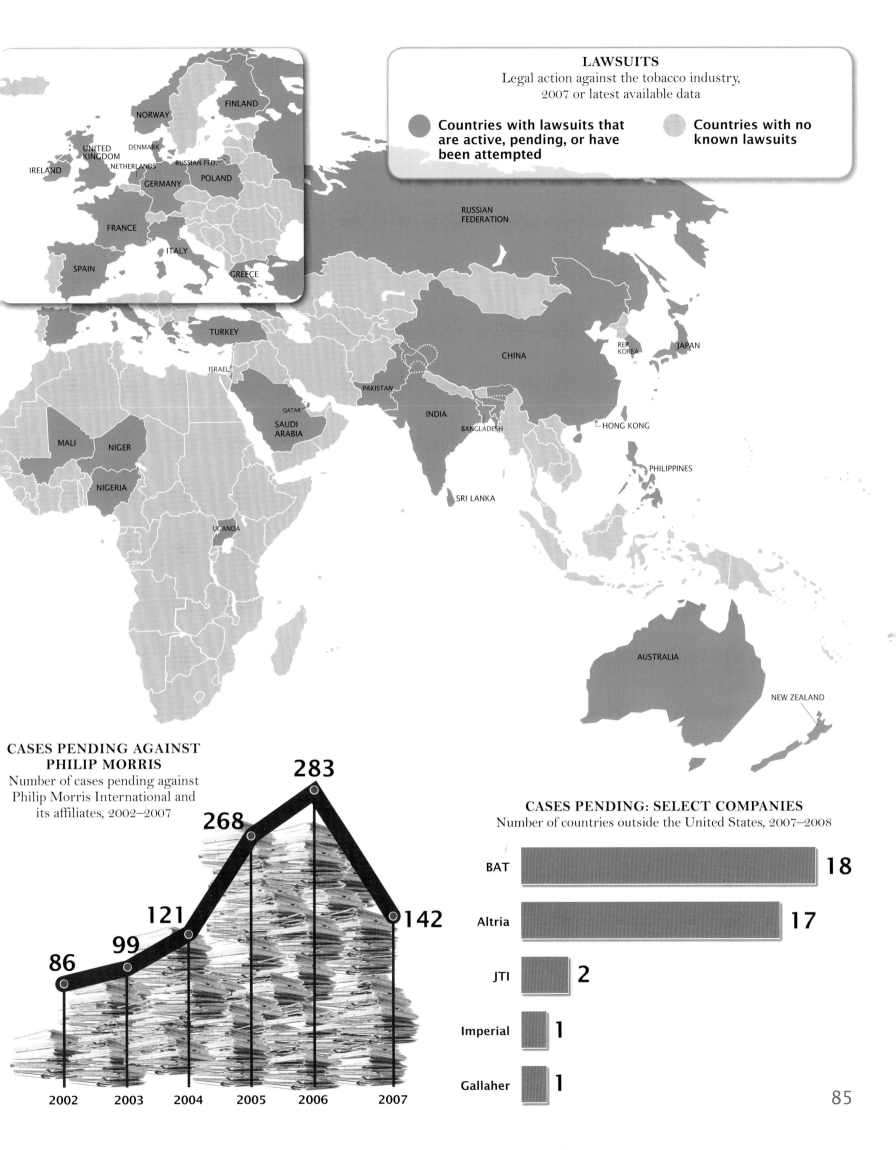

LAWSUITS
Legal action against the tobacco industry,
2007 or latest available data

● Countries with lawsuits that are active, pending, or have been attempted
○ Countries with no known lawsuits

CASES PENDING AGAINST PHILIP MORRIS

Number of cases pending against Philip Morris International and its affiliates, 2002–2007

86 — 2002
99 — 2003
121 — 2004
268 — 2005
283 — 2006
142 — 2007

CASES PENDING: SELECT COMPANIES

Number of countries outside the United States, 2007–2008

BAT — 18
Altria — 17
JTI — 2
Imperial — 1
Gallaher — 1

85

RELIGION

"Every human being is the author of his own health or disease."

—SIDDHÂRTHA GAUTAMA BUDDHA (563–483 BCE)

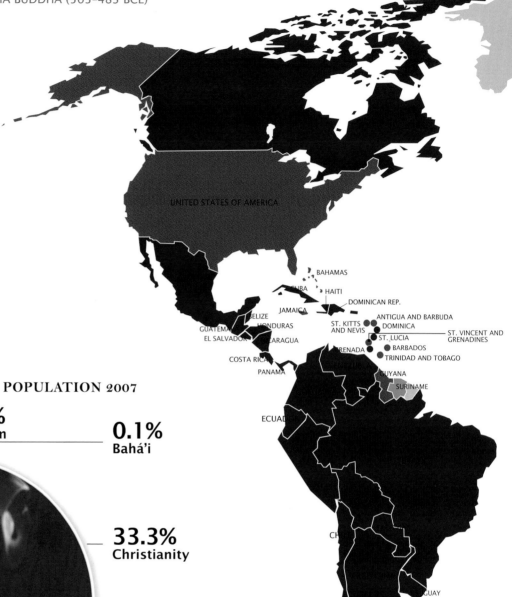

Religion plays an important role in the daily life of many people throughout the world, influencing each nation's social norms and cultural traditions.

Tobacco, an indigenous plant of the Americas, is considered a sacrament by many Native American cultures. In the Cherokee tradition, for instance, smoke acts as a messenger carrying prayers to the spirit world. In the pre-Columbian era, ceremonial and ritualistic uses of tobacco leaf in Native American culture were infrequent and typically did not lead to addiction or create public health problems. Today, however, Native American and indigenous groups exhibit some of the highest rates of tobacco use in the world.

Most major religions of the Old World, founded before the advent of the tobacco pandemic, do not specifically address tobacco in their founding texts, but the general precepts of every religion agree that people should protect their life and health, as well as the sanctity of their family and community.

RELIGIONS OF THE WORLD BY POPULATION 2007

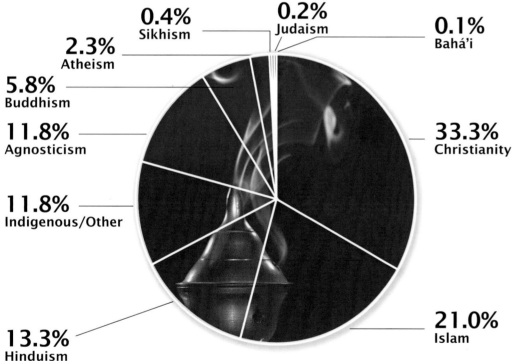

0.4% Sikhism

0.2% Judaism

0.1% Bahá'i

2.3% Atheism

5.8% Buddhism

11.8% Agnosticism

33.3% Christianity

11.8% Indigenous/Other

13.3% Hinduism

21.0% Islam

"Offering cigarettes to monks is a sin."

—Thai Anti-Smoking Campaign Project poster used to curb smoking among Buddhist monks, 2002

"Since the damage caused by smoking to human life is so evident, there is no doubt that it is haram (forbidden)."

—Dr. Ahmad Omar Hashim, Al-Azhar University, Cairo, Egypt

"If smoking causes substantial harm to a male or female smoker or to the fetus, then it is prohibited."

—Shiite Grand Ayatollah Ali Sistani, Najaf, Iraq

"Whatever short-lived pleasure it may provide, there is now no doubt that the use of tobacco is a cause of much disease and misery."

—His Holiness The 14th Dalai Lama

"Our faith traditions inform us that our bodies are gifts from God and, therefore, should be treasured and treated with dignity. This means, among other things, that tobacco companies should not be allowed to entice our children to pollute their bodies."

—James Winkler, chair, Faith United Against Tobacco Convention

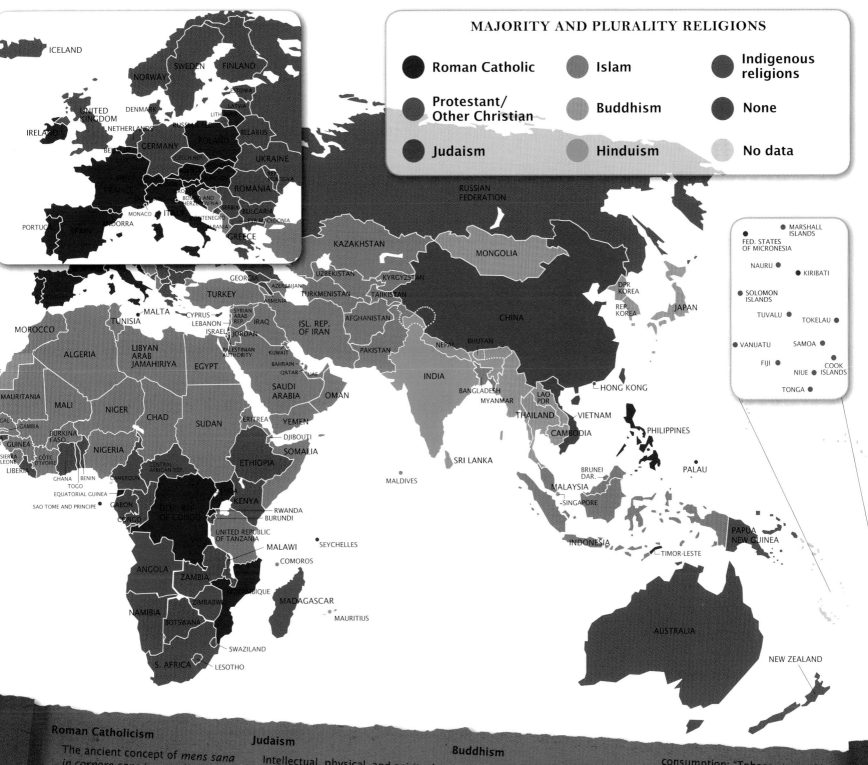

MAJORITY AND PLURALITY RELIGIONS

- ● Roman Catholic
- ● Protestant/Other Christian
- ● Judaism
- ● Islam
- ● Buddhism
- ● Hinduism
- ● Indigenous religions
- ● None
- ● No data

Roman Catholicism

The ancient concept of *mens sana in corpore sano* (a sound mind in a sound body) was reaffirmed in the Pontifical Council's recognition of tobacco's harmful effects and the papal committee's 2002 ban on public smoking in the Vatican.

Christianity

Many Christian churches consider tobacco a violation of the body— "the temple of the Holy Spirit." Churches may abjure tobacco in the interests of social justice and to achieve wholeness and well-being for their members and the broader community.

Judaism

Intellectual, physical, and spiritual faculties are considered gifts presented to each human. Striving to preserve the body is a measure of the esteem in which those gifts are held. Halakha—Jewish law—prohibits the smoking of tobacco products.

Islam

Islamic law (Fiqh) concerning the integrity of the individual proscribes all products and practices that jeopardize life or health. Because tobacco is harmful to health, its consumption is contrary to the spirit of Islam. In 2002, the two holy cities of Mecca and Medina in Saudi Arabia were declared tobacco-free.

Buddhism

Buddhism teaches the path to enlightenment, freedom, and mental clarity. Freedom implies no dependence or addiction. Anything that harms the body or mind, one's own or those of others, must be avoided.

Hinduism

Hinduism defines *vyasana* as a dependence unnecessary for the preservation of health. *Vyasana*—addiction—causes suffering and impedes attainment of a spiritual life. Tobacco use violates Hindu principles against causing harm to self and others.

Church of Jesus Christ of Latter-Day Saints (Mormons)

Mormon Prophet Joseph Smith specifically proscribed tobacco consumption: "Tobacco is not for the body, neither for the belly, and is not good for man . . ." (*Doctrine and Covenants* 89:4, 8). The state of Utah—70 percent Mormon—has the lowest smoking prevalence and lung cancer rates in the United States.

Bahá'i Faith

The Tablet on Purity scriptures by 'Abdu'l-Bahá condemns the use of tobacco and asks God to "Deliver [the people of Baha] from intoxicating drinks and tobacco, save them, rescue them. . . ."

Sikhism

The Reht Maryada (Code of Conduct) strictly forbids tobacco use, one of the four cardinal transgressions, or *Kurahits*.

CHAPTER 31

THE FUTURE

"In the 20th century, the tobacco epidemic killed 100 million people worldwide. During the 21st century, it could kill 1 billion."

—WORLD HEALTH ORGANIZATION MPOWER REPORT, 2008

Future predictions are by their nature speculative, but some things are certain: the tobacco pandemic, with its enormous health and economic costs, is both increasing and also shifting from developed to developing nations, with more women smoking than ever before.

The tobacco industry is consolidating and shifting focus from high-resource to low- and middle-resource countries, where there may be less government regulation and organized public opposition to the machinations of transnational tobacco companies.

The global tobacco pandemic is worse today than it was 50 years ago, and it will be even worse in another 50 years unless extraordinary efforts are made now. Even if smoking prevalence rates begin to decline, the number of smokers in the world will inexorably rise for the foreseeable future, due principally to world population growth.

Many countries, including low-resource countries, have shown that tobacco can be controlled and smoking rates can be reduced. These successes can be reproduced by any responsible nation, but only through concerted, comprehensive, and sustained governmental and community action. The future is uncertain, and some of the events predicted here may never occur. However, preventing youth initiation and encouraging cessation clearly require steadfast political will to tackle the tobacco industry and allocate appropriate resources proportional to the health and economic magnitude of the tobacco problem.

The means to curb this pandemic are clear and within reach.

2000–2010 | 2010–2020

Number of smokers, billions

◼ Number of smokers (assuming constant prevalence and medium variant projected population)

◻ Number of smokers (assuming reduced prevalence of -1.0% per year, medium variant projected population)

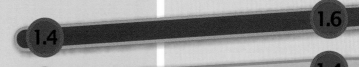

1.4   1.6

1.3   1.4

Health

Tobacco kills more than 5 million people annually and accounts for about 8.8% of all global deaths and 4.2% of disabilities.

Almost half the world's children are exposed to passive smoking.

Tobacco kills more than 6 million people annually, 50% more people than are killed by HIV/AIDS, and accounting for 10% of all global deaths.

Individuals genetically prone to nicotine addiction and tobacco-related diseases can be identified at birth.

Economics

Global annual economic costs (health-care costs plus costs to the economy) of tobacco: US$500 billion a year by 2010.

Tobacco-related illnesses become a leading health expenditure in many countries.

Most governments conclude that the economic costs of tobacco outstrip any revenues.

The Tobacco Industry

Attempts to produce genetically modified tobacco.

Some tobacco companies buy pharmaceutical companies.

The tobacco industry claims to be socially responsible.

Some tobacco companies support increased government regulation to protect their market share or other interests.

Industry consolidation leads to two to three huge conglomerates accounting for the bulk of global sales.

Niche markets increase (e.g., cigars, snuff, bidis, kretek).

Liberalization of global trade rules welcomed by the industry.

Smuggled cigarettes overtake legal sales.

The majority of tobacco products are non-combustible.

Industry introduces new innovative products that purportedly reduce harm.

Huge advances are made in genetics. The tobacco plant is harnessed to produce vaccines and other beneficial products.

Action Taken

The WHO Framework Convention on Tobacco Control (FCTC) is ratified by most countries.

Many countries ban smoking in all public places and workplaces.

In many countries, public perceptions shift against smoking, and nonsmoking becomes the norm.

Countries focus on implementation of the FCTC and its protocols.

New, less-hazardous tobacco products increase, posing a great challenge for smokers not to be misled in thinking these are safe.

The WHO publishes its second report on the global status of the tobacco epidemic.

Tobacco advertising and promotion are eliminated worldwide.

Vaccine is produced to switch off nicotine receptors.

Medical schools globally introduce systematic teaching on tobacco.

Smoke-free areas become the norm.

Cigarettes are packaged in plain black and white wrappers displaying only brand name and graphic warnings.

Economies with a large tobacco farming sector are assisted in diversifying crops.

Nicotine replacement therapy sold over the counter worldwide.

Incentives for quitting include monetary savings through rebates and lower health insurance premiums.

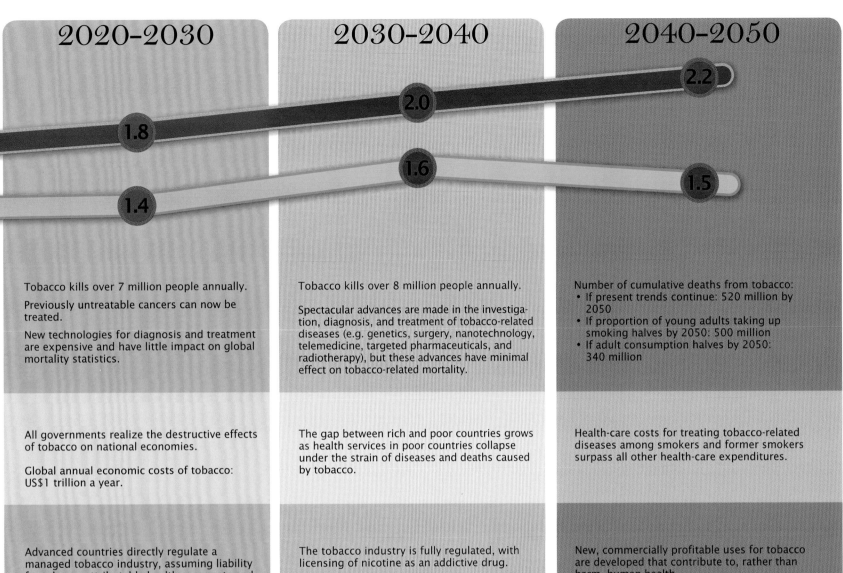

2020–2030

1.8

1.4

Tobacco kills over 7 million people annually.

Previously untreatable cancers can now be treated.

New technologies for diagnosis and treatment are expensive and have little impact on global mortality statistics.

All governments realize the destructive effects of tobacco on national economies.

Global annual economic costs of tobacco: US$1 trillion a year.

Advanced countries directly regulate a managed tobacco industry, assuming liability for tobacco-attributable health-care costs and other economic costs of tobacco.

Cigarettes available only by prescription in high-resource countries.

Continued trend in privatization absorbs remaining state-run tobacco companies.

Tobacco control funded from a percentage of tobacco tax in most countries.

Duty-free tobacco no longer exists.

Health education messages are more skillful and hard-hitting, and are disseminated more effectively.

In every country, the tax on tobacco is at least 75% of the retail price.

2030–2040

2.0

1.6

Tobacco kills over 8 million people annually.

Spectacular advances are made in the investigation, diagnosis, and treatment of tobacco-related diseases (e.g. genetics, surgery, nanotechnology, telemedicine, targeted pharmaceuticals, and radiotherapy), but these advances have minimal effect on tobacco-related mortality.

The gap between rich and poor countries grows as health services in poor countries collapse under the strain of diseases and deaths caused by tobacco.

The tobacco industry is fully regulated, with licensing of nicotine as an addictive drug.

Manufacture, promotion, and sale strictly controlled by government agencies.

World's top tobacco companies now based in Asia.

Virtually no tobacco is grown in the United States.

2040–2050

2.2

1.5

Number of cumulative deaths from tobacco:
• If present trends continue: 520 million by 2050
• If proportion of young adults taking up smoking halves by 2050: 500 million
• If adult consumption halves by 2050: 340 million

Health-care costs for treating tobacco-related diseases among smokers and former smokers surpass all other health-care expenditures.

New, commercially profitable uses for tobacco are developed that contribute to, rather than harm, human health.

The future is uncertain. Some of these events may never occur.

CHAPTER 32

HISTORY OF TOBACCO

6000 BCE–2009 CE

6000 BCE
Americas First cultivation of the tobacco plant.

circa 1 BCE
Americas Indigenous Americans began smoking and using tobacco enemas.

Americas Huron Indian myth: "In ancient times, when the land was barren and the people were starving, the Great Spirit sent forth a woman to save humanity. As she traveled over the world everywhere her right hand touched the soil, there grew potatoes. And everywhere her left hand touched the soil, there grew corn. And in the place where she had sat, there grew tobacco."

1492
Christopher Columbus and his crew returned to Europe from the Americas with the first tobacco leaves and seeds ever seen on the continent. A crew member, Rodrigo de Jerez, was seen smoking and imprisoned by the Inquisition, which believed he was possessed by the devil.

Early 1500s
Middle East Tobacco introduced when the Turks took it to Egypt.

1530–1600
China Tobacco introduced via Japan or the Philippines.

1558
Europe Tobacco plant brought to Europe. Attempts at cultivation failed.

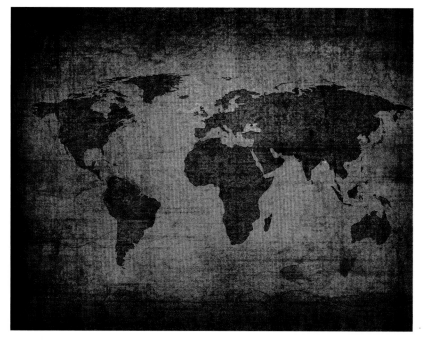

1560
Africa Portuguese and Spanish traders introduced tobacco to Africa.

1560
France Diplomat Jean Nicot, Lord of Villemain, introduced tobacco from Portugal. Queen Catherine de Medici used it to treat her migraines.

1577
Europe European doctors recommended tobacco as a cure for toothache, falling fingernails, worms, halitosis, lockjaw, and cancer.

1592–1598
Korea The Japanese Army introduced tobacco into Korea.

circa 1600
India Tobacco first introduced.

1603
Japan Use of tobacco well-established.

1604
England King James I wrote *A Counterblaste to Tobacco.* "Smoking is a custom loathsome to the eye, hateful to the nose, harmful to the brain, dangerous to the lungs, and in the black, stinking fume thereof nearest resembling the horrible Stygian smoke of the pit that is bottomless."

1600s
China Philosopher Fang Yizhi pointed out that long years of smoking "scorches one's lung."

1608–1609
Japan Ban on smoking introduced to prevent fires.

1612
Americas Tobacco first grown commercially.

1614
England 7,000 tobacco shops opened with the first sale of Virginia tobacco.

1633
Turkey Death penalty imposed for smoking.

1634
China Qing Dynasty decreed a smoking ban during which a violator was executed. This was not to protect health, but to address the inequality of trade with Korea.

1650s
South Africa European settlers grew tobacco and used it as a form of currency.

1692 and 1717
Korea Bans on smoking in Choson introduced to reduce fire risk.

circa 1710
Russia Peter the Great encouraged his courtiers to smoke tobacco and drink coffee, which was seen as fashionable and pro-European.

1700s
Africa/Americas African slaves forced to work in tobacco fields.

1719
France Smoking was prohibited in many places.

1753
Sweden Botanist Carolus Linnaeus named the plant genus nicotiana and describes two species, *nicotiana rustica* and *nicotiana tabacum.*

1761
England First study of the effects of tobacco by Dr. John Hill; snuff

users were warned they risked nasal cancers.

1769

New Zealand Captain James Cook arrived smoking a pipe, and was promptly doused in case he was a demon.

1771

France French official was condemned to be hanged for admitting foreign tobacco into the country.

1788

Australia Tobacco arrived with the First Fleet, eleven ships which sailed from England carrying mostly convicts and crew.

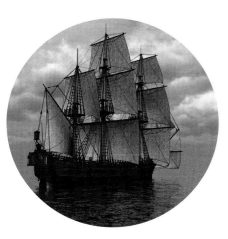

1795

Sammuel Thomas von Soemmering reported cancers of the lip in pipe smokers.

18th century

Snuff was the most popular mode of tobacco use.

1800

Canada Tobacco first grown commercially.

1833

UK Phosphorus friction matches introduced on a commercial scale, making smoking more convenient.

1840

France Frederic Chopin's mistress, the Baroness de Dudevant, likely to have been the first woman to smoke in public (in Paris).

1847

England Philip Morris Esq, a tobacconist and importer of fine cigars, opened a shop in London selling hand-rolled Turkish cigarettes.

1854

England Philip Morris began making his own cigarettes. Old Bond Street soon became the center of the retail tobacco trade.

1858

China Treaty of Tianjin allowed cigarettes to be imported into China duty-free.

1862

USA First federal tobacco tax was introduced to help finance the Civil War.

1876

Korea Foreign cigarettes and matches were introduced.

1880s

England Richard Benson and William Hedges opened a tobacconist shop near Philip Morris in London.

1881

USA First practical cigarette-making machine patented by James Bonsack. It could produce 120,000 cigarettes a day, each machine doing the work of 48 people. Production costs plummeted, and—with the invention of the safety match a few decades later—cigarette-smoking began its explosive growth.

circa 1890s

Indonesia Clove cigarette, the kretek, invented.

before 1900

Lung cancer was extremely rare.

1901–02

England Imperial Tobacco Company Limited (ITL) and British American Tobacco (BAT) were founded.

1903

Brazil Tobacco company Souza Cruz founded.

1913

USA Birth of the "modern" cigarette: RJ Reynolds introduced the Camel brand.

1915

Japan Cancer was induced in laboratory animals for the first time by applying coal tar to rabbits' skin at Tokyo University.

1921

Korea Korea Ginseng Corporation became Korea Tobacco and Ginseng (KTG) and a monopoly was formed.

1924

Philip Morris introduced Marlboro as a women's cigarette as "mild as May."

1924

Reader's Digest published "Does Tobacco Injure the Human Body," the beginning of a *Reader's Digest* campaign to make people think before starting to smoke.

1929

USA Edward Bernays mounted a "freedom march" of smoking debutantes/fashion models who walk down Fifth Avenue in New York during the Easter parade dressed as Statues of Liberty and holding aloft their Lucky Strike cigarettes as "torches of freedom."

1929

Germany Fritz Lickint of Dresden published the first formal statistical evidence of a lung cancer-tobacco link, based on a case series showing that lung cancer sufferers were likely to be smokers.

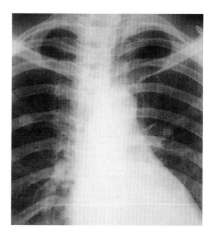

1936

Germany Fritz Lickint first used the term "Passivrauchen" (passive smoking) in Tabakgenuss und Gesundheit.

1939

USA Tobacco companies found price-fixing.

1939

USA Drs. Alton Ochsner and Michael DeBakey first reported the association of smoking and lung cancer.

1947

Canada Dr. Norman Delarue compared 50 patients with lung cancer with 50 patients hospitalized with other diseases. He discovered that over 90 percent of the first group—but only half of the second—were smokers, and confidently predicted that by 1950 no one would be smoking.

1950

USA The link between smoking and lung cancer was confirmed. A landmark article "Tobacco smoking as a possible etiologic factor in bronchogenic carcinoma" by E. L. Wynder and Evarts Graham was published in *The Journal of the American Medical Association.* The same issue featured a full-page ad for Chesterfields with the actress Gene Tierney and golfer Ben Hogan; the journal accepted tobacco ads until 1953.

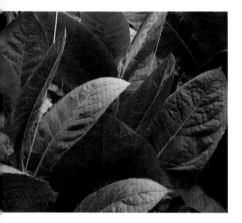

1951
UK Dr. Richard Doll and Prof. Austin Bradford Hill conducted the first large-scale case control study on the link between smoking and lung cancer.

1953
USA Tobacco executives met in New York City to find a way to deal with recent scientific data pointing to the health hazards of cigarettes.

1950s
China State monopoly takes control of the tobacco business, and foreign tobacco companies left China. BAT, almost half of whose revenues came from China, was especially hurt.

1954
USA St. Louis factory worker Ira C. Lowe filed the first product liability action against a tobacco company on behalf of her smoker husband, who died from cancer. The tobacco company won.

1954
USA The Marlboro cowboy was created for Philip Morris by Chicago ad agency Leo Burnett.

1954
USA Tobacco Industry Research Committee (TIRC) placed a nationwide two-page ad: "A frank statement to cigarette smokers."

1957
Vatican Pope Pius XII suggested that the Jesuit order give up smoking.

1958
USA Tobacco Institute formed.

1960
USA Framingham Heart Study found cigarette smoking increased the risk of heart disease.

1962
UK First Report of the Royal College of Physicians of London on Smoking and Health.

1963
World Tobacco and *Tobacco Journal International*, tobacco industry trade journals, first published.

1964
USA First US Surgeon General's report on smoking and health announced that smoking caused lung cancer in men.

1965
WHO established the International Agency for Research on Cancer (IARC) based in Lyons, France.

1965
UK Cigarette advertising on TV was banned.

1967
USA First World Conference on Tobacco or Health held in New York.

1969
USA Surgeon General's Report confirmed the link between maternal smoking and low birth weight.

1971
UK ASH UK established the first national tobacco control organization.

1971
USA Cigarette manufacturers first agreed to put health warnings on advertisements. This agreement was later made law.

1972
Marlboro became the bestselling cigarette in the world.

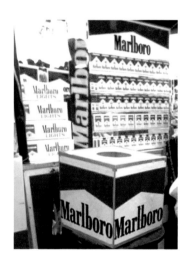

1972
International Association for the Study of Lung Cancer was inaugurated.

1974
France Joe Camel was born—used in French poster campaign for Camel cigarettes.

1976
USA Shimp v. New Jersey Bell Telephone Co. filed the world's first lawsuit regarding second-hand smoke. The office worker was granted an injunction to ensure a smoke-free area in her workplace.

1977
Italy The Martignacco Project community prevention trial resulted in a reduction of coronary heart disease.

1977
USA First Great American Smokeout held nationally, during which smokers quit smoking on the third Thursday of November.

1978
Australia The three-year community study North Coast Healthy Lifestyle Programme showed a significant reduction in smoking.

1978
USA A Roper Report prepared for the Tobacco Institute concluded that the nonsmokers' rights movement was "the most dangerous development to the viability of the tobacco industry that has yet occurred."

1979
USA Tobacco Control Resource Center and its Tobacco Products Liability Project were formed.

1979
The Freedom Organization for the Right to Enjoy Smoking Tobacco (FOREST) formed.

1979
Australia Activist group BUGAUP (Billboard Utilising Graffitists Against Unhealthy

Promotions) was formed, re-facing tobacco and alcohol billboards.

1981

Japan Professor Takeshi Hirayama (1923–1995) published the first report linking passive smoking and lung cancer in the nonsmoking wives of men who smoked.

1983

Europe ERC Group plc, an independent market research group, published first European Tobacco Market Report.

1984

Nicotine gum was first introduced.

1985

USA Lung cancer surpassed breast cancer as number-one cancer killer of women.

by 1985

73 percent of the world's tobacco was grown in developing countries.

1987

USA Smoke-free Educational Services founded, advocating the right of all employees to work in a safe, healthy, smoke-free environment.

1988

First WHO report on the effects of smokeless tobacco.

1988

USA Framingham Heart Study found cigarette smoking increased the risk of stroke.

1988

First WHO World No Tobacco Day, subsequently an annual event on May 31, with different annual themes and awards of commemorative medals.

1989

Asia The Asia Pacific Association for the Control of Tobacco (APACT) was established by Dr. David Yen of the John Tung Foundation, Taiwan, China.

1990

GLOBALink inaugurated, the international interactive Web site and marketplace founded by the International Union Against Cancer for the international tobacco-control community.

1990

Tobacco Control in the Third World: A Resource Atlas was released.

1990

International Network of Women Against Tobacco (INWAT) formed.

1990

China Chinese Association on Smoking and Health inaugurated.

1991

UK International Agency on Tobacco and Health (IATH) formed to act as an information and advisory service for the least-developed countries.

1991

Realization that chemicals in cigarette smoke switch on a gene that makes lung cells vulnerable to the chemicals' cancer-causing properties.

1991

International Network Towards Smoke-free Hospitals inaugurated, aiming to give healthy environment to hospital staff and patients.

1992

Tobacco Control journal founded by the British Medical Journals group. This was the first international peer-reviewed journal on tobacco control, and in 2004, the journal had the highest impact factor of all in the substance abuse field.

1992

Northern Ireland, UK First conference on women and tobacco initiated by the UICC (International Union Against Cancer), the Ulster Cancer Foundation, and the Health Promotion Agency of Northern Ireland.

1993

USA Environmental Protection Agency (EPA) declared cigarette smoke a Class-A carcinogen.

1993

South Africa Tobacco Products Control Amendment Act passed.

1993

Europe European Network on Young People and Tobacco (ENYPAT) founded.

1994

USA Cigarette executives testified before Congress that in their opinion nicotine was not addictive.

1994

Society for Research on Nicotine and Tobacco founded.

1994

USA Confidential internal tobacco industry documents leaked to Professor Stan Glantz.

1994

Austria First TABEXPO held in Vienna. TABEXPO stages exhibitions and congresses for the international tobacco industry.

1994

International Non Governmental Coalition Against Tobacco (INGCAT) founded.

1994

First international "Quit & Win" campaign.

1994

Canada Research for International Tobacco Control (RITC) inaugurated, with a major focus on developing countries.

1994

USA State of Mississippi filed first lawsuit by a health authority for reimbursement of money expended to treat smokers with smoking-caused illnesses. It ended with an out-of-court settlement.

1995

USA Smokescreen.org (later Smoke-free.net) was inaugurated. Focusing on the right to breathe clean air, this was the first Web-based advocacy site that enabled

1995–2009

visitors to send faxes directly to their elected officials. Mainly used by Americans, but also by 10,000 international participants.

1995
Italy The Bellagio statement on tobacco and sustainable development was issued by members of retreat at Rockefeller Foundation's Bellagio Study and Conference Centre.

1995
International Council of Nurses (ICN) published position statement on tobacco.

1995
USA Federal Drug Administration declared cigarettes to be "drug delivery devices." Restrictions were proposed on marketing and sales to reduce smoking by young people.

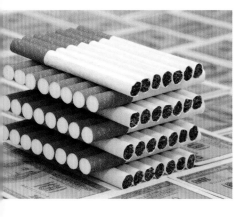

1990s
Cigars became fashionable again.

1995
Forces International (Fight Ordinances and Restrictions to Control and Eliminate Smoking), an ostensibly grassroots pro-tobacco organization unaffiliated with the tobacco industry, established.

1995
USA "Marlboro Man" David McLean died of lung cancer.

1996
USA First smoking cessation guideline, issued by the Public Health Service, Federal Government.

1997
Europe European Network for Smoking Prevention (ENSP) created.

1997
Scotland, UK Doctors and Tobacco: Tobacco Control Resource Centre (TCRC) formed by the European Forum Medical Associations (EFMA). The TCRC is based at the British Medical Association in Edinburgh, and works in partnership with national medical associations across Europe.

1997
USA Congress passed a bill prohibiting the Departments of State, Justice, and Commerce from promoting the sale or export of tobacco.

1998
Studies confirmed the harmfulness of smoking fewer than 10 cigarettes a day.

1998
WHO's Tobacco-free Initiative (TFI) was established.

1998
United Nations Foundation first funded a tobacco control project.

1998
Australia Tobacco Control Supersite Web site inaugurated, enabling exploration of internal, previously private tobacco industry documents, and providing access to a wide range of information relevant to smoking prevention and control in Australia.

1998
USA Master Settlement Agreement among Attorneys General of 46 states and five territories with tobacco companies to settle lawsuits.

1999
USA Network for Accountability of Tobacco Transnationals (NATT) founded by Infact, made up of environmental, consumers, human rights, and corporate accountability organizations working together to forge new ground in international law to prevent life-threatening abuses by transnational corporations.

1999
Global Youth Tobacco Surveys (GYTS) commenced.

1999
World Bank report: *Curbing the Epidemic: Governments and the Economics of Tobacco Control.*

1999
Sweden Swedish International Development Cooperation Agency (Sida) first supported tobacco control projects.

1999
UK Britain's royal family ordered the removal of its seal of approval and royal crest from Gallaher's Benson and Hedges cigarettes by 2000.

1999
USA US Justice Department sued the tobacco industry to recover billions of government dollars spent on smoking-related health-care, accusing cigarette makers of "fraud and deceit."

2000
Framework Convention Alliance (FCA) of NGOs formed to support the WHO Framework Convention on Tobacco Control (FCTC) and related protocols.

2000
USA First Luther L. Terry Awards for contributions to tobacco control.

2000
Global Partnerships for Tobacco Control founded by Essential Action to help support and strengthen international tobacco control activities at the grassroots level.

2000
International Tobacco Evidence Network (ITEN) established, with the goal of expanding global research.

2000
Rockefeller Foundation International Health Research Awards for "Trading Tobacco for Health" in selected ASEAN countries.

2000
South Africa Tobacco Products Control Amendment Act came into effect, strictly regulating smoking and advertising.

2001
Southeast Asia Tobacco Control Alliance (SEATCA) formed to

act as supportive base for government and nongovernment tobacco control workers and advocates.

2001
USA A new report, *Clearing the Smoke: Assessing the Science Base for Tobacco Harm Reduction*, from the Institute of Medicine (IOM) was released.

2001
WHO published *Tobacco & the Rights of the Child*.

2001
Czech Republic Philip Morris released a report to the government that concluded that smokers save the state money—by dying early.

2002
TobaccoPedia, the online tobacco encyclopedia, was inaugurated.

2002
USA Global Tobacco Research Network founded by the Institute for Global Tobacco Control at Johns Hopkins University.

2002
WHO published the first edition of *The Tobacco Atlas*.

2002
USA Fogarty International Centre, National Institutes of Health, allocated funding for tobacco research projects.

2003
World Medical Association launched "The Doctors' Manifesto for Global Tobacco Control."

2003
Treatobacco Web-based database and educational resource for treatment of tobacco dependence established by the Society for Research on Nicotine and Tobacco.

2003
The Global Network of Pharmacists Against Tobacco launched.

2004
Ireland Workplace smoking ban, including pubs and restaurants, implemented. Exactly one year after the ban, cigarette sales had declined by 18 percent.

2004
First general textbook for health professionals on tobacco published: *Tobacco: Science, Policy and Public Health*.

2004
Europe The EU Commission published the ASPECT report, Tobacco or Health in the European Union: Past, Present and Future, the first comprehensive overview of tobacco control in the 25 EU member countries plus Norway, Iceland, and Switzerland.

2004
Uganda Environment Minister Kahinda Otafiire announced a ban on smoking in restaurants, educational institutions, and bars.

2004
Canada Non-Smokers' Rights Association, founded in 1974, the first such association, celebrated its 30th anniversary.

2004
Myriad Editions created interactive Internet mapping of *The Tobacco Atlas* launched by Global Tobacco Research Network, Johns Hopkins University.

2004
WHO's "Code of practice on tobacco control for health professional organizations" launched.

2004
IARC Monograph on Tobacco Smoke and Involuntary Smoking released, conclusively refuting extensive tobacco industry disinformation.

2004
India Complete ban on tobacco advertising and promotions came into effect.

2005
World Dental Federation (FDI) launches Tobacco or Oral Health publication.

2005
WHO Framework Convention on Tobacco Control (FCTC) came into force, using international law to reduce tobacco use. This convention was initiated by Ruth Roemer in 1993.

2006
Second edition of *The Tobacco Atlas* published by American Cancer Society in print and online at www.tobaccoresearch.net/atlas.

2006
Bloomberg Global Initiative to Reduce Tobacco Use in low- and middle-income countries launched

with $125 million donation from Michael Bloomberg, mayor of New York City.

2008
The Global Smokefree Partnership formed to promote effective smoke-free air policies worldwide.

2008
The first WHO MPOWER report on the global status of the tobacco epidemic published.

2008
Bill & Melinda Gates Foundation pledges $125 million to global tobacco control. Michael Bloomberg pledges an additional $250 million to the Bloomberg Global Initiative, bringing total outlay to $500 million over seven years, 2006–2013.

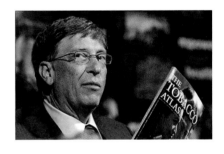

2009
Third edition of *The Tobacco Atlas* published by the American Cancer Society and World Lung Foundation.

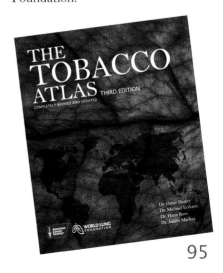

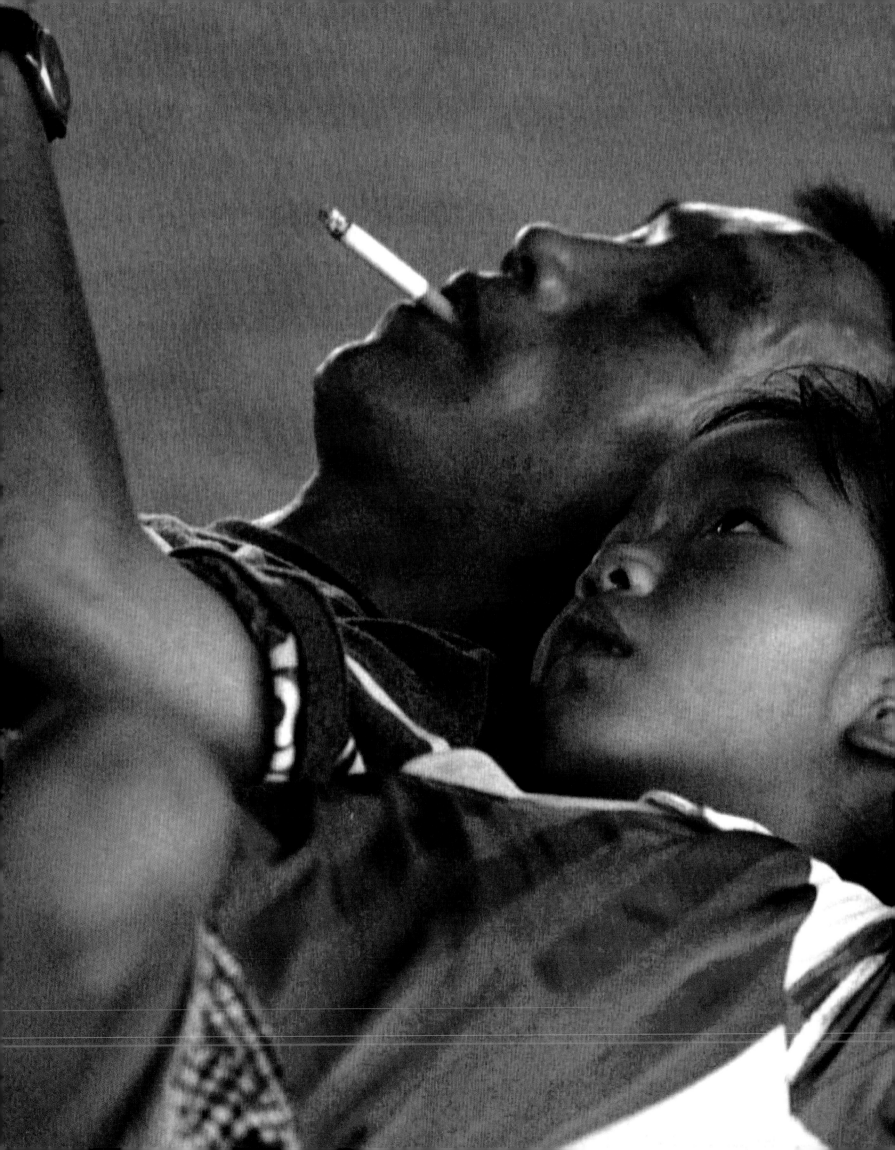

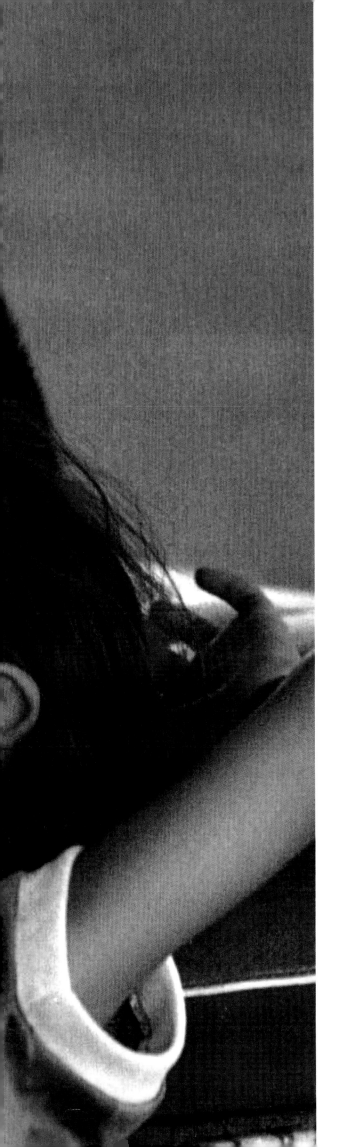

PART SIX

WORLD TABLES

"An apple a day keeps the doctor away, but when tobacco smells like an apple it can be injurious to health."

— Bombay High Court, which upheld Brihanmumbai Municipal Corporation's decision to ban hookah parlors in Mumbai.

TABLE A THE DEMOGRAPHICS OF TOBACCO

| COUNTRY | 1 Population | 2 Adult Smoking Prevalence—Male (percentages) | | | | | | | |
| | | Male Age Standardized | | Male Crude | | | | | |
	(thousands)	Current Cigarette Use	Current Any Tobacco Use	Current Tobacco Use	Current Tobacco Smoking	Daily Tobacco Smoking	Current Cigarette Use	Daily Cigarette Use	Age Range
AFGHANISTAN	32,738	-	-	82.0	-	-	-	-	18+
ALBANIA	3,172	40.5	40.5	-	-	-	46.3	-	15–49
ALGERIA	33,351	26.6	29.9	-	38.1	32.3	-	-	25–64
ANDORRA	67	36.5	36.5	-	42.0	-	-	-	16+
ANGOLA	16,557	-	-	-	-	-	-	-	-
ANTIGUA AND BARBUDA	84	-	-	-	-	-	-	-	-
ARGENTINA	39,134	34.3	34.6	-	-	-	35.1	26.2	18+
ARMENIA	3,010	55.1	55.1	-	-	-	60.5	-	15–49
AUSTRALIA	20,701	-	-	-	-	-	-	16.6	14+
AUSTRIA	8,281	46.4	46.4	-	48.0	40.2	-	-	14–99
AZERBAIJAN	8,484	-	-	-	-	-	-	-	-
BAHAMAS	327	-	-	-	19.3	-	-	-	16–59
BAHRAIN	739	25.6	26.1	-	15.0	-	-	-	15+
BANGLADESH	155,990	42.8	47.0	48.6	41.0	-	-	-	15+
BARBADOS	293	16.9	18.4	-	19.3	-	-	-	15+
BELARUS	9,733	63.7	63.7	-	56.8	-	-	-	16+
BELGIUM	10,541	30.1	30.1	-	32.5	28.0	-	-	15+
BELIZE	298	-	-	-	-	-	-	-	-
BENIN	8,760	-	-	-	-	-	-	-	-
BHUTAN	649	-	-	10.0	-	-	-	-	Adult
BOLIVIA	9,354	33.8	34.1	-	-	-	-	-	-
BOSNIA AND HERZEGOVINA	3,926	49.3	49.3	-	54.2	46.6	-	-	18+
BOTSWANA	1,858	-	-	-	-	-	-	-	-
BRAZIL	189,320	-	-	-	20.3	16.9	-	-	18+
BRUNEI DARUSSALAM	382	-	-	-	-	-	-	-	-
BULGARIA	7,693	47.5	47.5	-	-	40.8	-	-	15+
BURKINA FASO	14,359	14.2	22.0	-	23.6	19.0	-	-	18+
BURUNDI	8,173	-	-	-	15.6	-	-	-	19+
CAMBODIA	14,197	37.9	40.5	-	-	54.0	-	-	18–64
CAMEROON	18,175	9.9	12.6	-	-	-	-	-	-
CANADA	32,649	19.0	-	-	-	-	19.9	15.3	15+
CAPE VERDE	519	-	-	-	-	-	-	-	-
CENTRAL AFRICAN REPUBLIC	4,265	-	-	-	-	-	-	-	-
CHAD	10,468	12.7	16.0	-	17.4	13.2	-	-	18+
CHILE	16,433	41.7	42.1	-	-	-	43.6	-	15+
CHINA	1,311,800	59.5	59.5	-	-	-	57.4	-	15–69
COLOMBIA	45,558	-	-	-	-	26.8	-	-	18–69
COMOROS	614	22.7	27.7	-	27.8	24.1	-	-	18+
CONGO	3,689	9.8	12.1	-	13.0	10.7	-	-	18+
CONGO, DEMOCRATIC REPUBLIC OF	60,644	10.9	13.5	-	14.2	10.2	-	-	15+
COOK ISLANDS	12	36.1	36.1	-	47.0	38.0	-	-	25–64
COSTA RICA	4,399	26.1	26.1	-	23.3	-	-	-	12–70
COTE D'IVOIRE	18,914	11.8	15.4	-	19.3	14.5	-	-	18+
CROATIA	4,441	38.9	38.9	-	31.6	30.0	-	-	18+
CUBA	11,267	36.1	43.4	-	-	41.6	-	-	15+
CYPRUS	771	-	-	-	-	38.1	-	-	15+
CZECH REPUBLIC	10,270	36.6	36.6	-	-	-	33.8	29.6	15+
DENMARK	5,437	36.1	36.1	-	31.5	28.6	-	-	15+

Female Age Standardized		Female Crude						Student Health Professionals' Smoking Prevalence	Youth Smoking Prevalence		Secondhand Smoking: Youth exposed in home	Cigarette Consumption	
								(percentages)	(percentages national data)		(percentages)	(annual per capita)	COUNTRY
Current Cigarette Use	Current Any Tobacco Use	Current Tobacco Use	Current Tobacco Smoking	Daily Tobacco Smoking	Current Cigarette Use	Daily Cigarette Use	Age Range		Boys	Girls			
-	-	17.0	-	-	-	-	18+	-	10.8	0.9	41.4	-	AFGHANISTAN
4.0	4.0	-	-	-	3.0	-	15-44	43.0	11.9	5.8	84.8	1,201	ALBANIA
0.2	0.3	-	0.5	0.4	-	-	25-64	-	-	-	-	577	ALGERIA
29.2	29.2	-	30.0	-	-	-	16+	-	44.9	46.8	-	-	ANDORRA
-	-	-	-	-	-	-		-	-	-	-	397	ANGOLA
-	-	-	-	-	-	-		-	2.7	4.4	18.9	-	ANTIGUA AND BARBUDA
23.5	25.4	-	-	-	24.9	18.6	18+	36.0	-	-	71.0	1,014	ARGENTINA
3.7	3.7	-	-	-	1.7	-	15-49	20.0	10.3	0.9	90.4	2,083	ARMENIA
-	-	-	-	-	-	15.2	14+	16.0	7	7	17.2	1,130	AUSTRALIA
40.1	40.1	-	47.0	35.5	-	-	14-99	-	26.1	37.1	-	1,684	AUSTRIA
0.9	0.9	-	-	-	0.6	-	15-44	-	-	-	-	1,089	AZERBAIJAN
-	-	-	3.8	-	-	-	16-59	-	6.2	3.7	21.6	-	BAHAMAS
2.4	2.9	-	3.1	-	-	-	15+	-	17.5	3.9	-	-	BAHRAIN
0.9	3.8	25.4	1.8	-	-	-	15+	28.0	-	-	34.3	172	BANGLADESH
2.3	3.0	-	3.0	-	-	-	15+	-	7.6	6.4	-	-	BARBADOS
21.1	21.1	-	15.4	-	-	-	16+	-	31.2	21.7	75.3	1,846	BELARUS
24.1	24.1	-	23.0	19.7	-	-	15+	-	23.1	23.8	-	1,763	BELGIUM
-	-	-	-	-	-	-		-	20.2	11.1	15.5	-	BELIZE
-	-	-	-	-	-	-		-	-	-	22.0	-	BENIN
-	-	7.0	-	-	-	-	adult	-	18.3	6.3	32.8	-	BHUTAN
26.1	29.2	-	32.5	-	29.6	-	15-49	41.0	-	-	35.6	178	BOLIVIA
35.1	35.1	-	34.2	24.9	-	-	18+	47.0	15.0	8.4	96.7	2,145	BOSNIA AND HERZEGOVINA
-	-	-	-	-	-	-		-	8.7	2.6	-	-	BOTSWANA
-	-	-	12.8	10.0	-	-	18+	17.0	-	-	37.2	580	BRAZIL
-	-	-	-	-	-	-		-	-	-	-	-	BRUNEI DARUSSALAM
27.8	27.8	-	-	22.8	-	-	15+	-	26.0	39.4	-	2,437	BULGARIA
0.8	11.2	-	11.1	10.3	-	-	18+	-	19.8	3.4	35.7	-	BURKINA FASO
-	-	-	11.4	-	-	-	19+	-	-	-	-	-	BURUNDI
5.7	6.5	-	6.0	-	-	-	18-64	-	4.6	0.2	47.0	447	CAMBODIA
1.3	2.2	-	-	-	-	-		-	-	-	-	141	CAMEROON
17.5	-	-	-	-	15.5	11.8	15+	12.0	10.5	9.0	-	897	CANADA
-	-	-	-	-	-	-		-	-	-	-	-	CAPE VERDE
-	-	-	-	-	-	-		-	-	-	-	-	CENTRAL AFRICAN REPUBLIC
1.0	2.6	-	2.9	2.1	-	-	18+	-	-	-	-	-	CHAD
30.5	33.6	-	-	-	31.8	-	15+	-	-	-	60.6	909	CHILE
3.7	3.7	-	-	-	2.6	-	15-69	6.0	-	-	47.0	1,646	CHINA
-	-	-	-	11.3	-	-	18-69	26.0	-	-	-	479	COLOMBIA
5.0	13.5	-	17.0	15.0	-	-	18+	-	13.5	6.9	39.3	-	COMOROS
0.4	1.0	-	1.3	1.1	-	-	18+	-	15.0	8.1	25.7	-	CONGO
0.6	2.6	-	1.2	0.6	-	-	15+	-	-	-	-	131	CONGO, DEMOCRATIC REPUBLIC OF
20.0	20.0	-	41.0	29.0	-	-	25-64	-	39.9	49.6	57.2	-	COOK ISLANDS
7.3	7.3	-	8.2	-	-	-	12-70	-	15.7	16.8	-	552	COSTA RICA
0.6	2.4	-	2.3	1.2	-	-	18+	-	-	-	44.2	198	COTE D'IVOIRE
29.1	29.1	-	22.9	17.8	-	-	18+	37.0	21.7	25.6	92.2	1,849	CROATIA
26.4	28.3	-	-	23.0	-	-	15+	-	11.2	8.8	61.4	1,010	CUBA
-	-	-	-	10.5	-	-	15+	-	12.3	8.2	87.0	1,830	CYPRUS
25.4	25.4	-	-	-	22.9	19.4	15+	22.0	29.8	32.7	37.6	2,368	CZECH REPUBLIC
30.6	30.6	-	25.9	24.1	-	-	15+	-	16.7	21.0	-	1,495	DENMARK

TABLE A THE DEMOGRAPHICS OF TOBACCO

| COUNTRY | 1 Population (thousands) | 2 Adult Smoking Prevalence—Male (percentages) | | | | | | | |
| | | Male Age Standardized | | Male Crude | | | | | |
		Current Cigarette Use	Current Any Tobacco Use	Current Tobacco Use	Current Tobacco Smoking	Daily Tobacco Smoking	Current Cigarette Use	Daily Cigarette Use	Age Range
DJIBOUTI	819	-	-	-	75.0	-	-	-	13+
DOMINICA	72	-	-	-	-	-	-	-	-
DOMINICAN REPUBLIC	9,615	15.7	17.5	-	17.2	15.3	-	-	18+
ECUADOR	13,202	23.6	23.9	-	26.3	6.1	-	-	18+
EGYPT	74,166	24.5	28.7	-	59.3	39.2	-	-	18+
EL SALVADOR	6,762	-	-	21.5	-	-	-	-	12–64
EQUATORIAL GUINEA	496	-	-	-	-	-	-	-	-
ERITREA	4,692	15.6	16.9	-	-	-	-	-	-
ESTONIA	1,342	49.9	49.9	-	55.5	47.7	-	-	16–64
ETHIOPIA	77,154	6.9	7.6	-	6.3	5.3	-	-	18+
FIJI	833	23.6	23.6	-	-	26.0	-	-	15–85
FINLAND	5,266	31.8	31.8	-	32.9	26.0	-	-	15–64
FRANCE	61,257	36.6	36.6	-	33.3	28.2	-	-	12–75
GABON	1,311	-	-	-	-	-	-	-	-
GAMBIA	1,663	17.2	29.3	-	38.5	-	-	-	15+
GEORGIA	4,433	57.1	57.1	-	58.1	50.4	-	-	18+
GERMANY	82,375	-	-	34.8	-	-	-	-	18+
GHANA	23,008	7.1	10.2	-	9.0	6.2	-	-	18+
GREECE	11,147	63.6	63.6	-	-	-	51.0	47.4	18–89
GRENADA	108	-	-	-	-	-	-	-	-
GUATEMALA	13,029	24.5	24.5	-	23.9	8.3	-	-	18+
GUINEA	9,181	-	-	-	-	-	-	-	-
GUINEA-BISSAU	1,646	-	-	-	-	-	-	-	-
GUYANA	739	-	-	-	-	-	-	-	-
HAITI	9,446	-	-	-	-	-	-	-	-
HONDURAS	6,969	-	-	-	-	-	-	-	-
HONG KONG SAR, CHINA	6,857	-	-	-	-	-	-	22.0	15+
HUNGARY	10,067	45.7	45.7	-	42.5	38.6	-	-	18+
ICELAND	302	26.1	26.1	-	22.0	19.3	-	-	15–89
INDIA	1,109,800	27.6	33.1	57.0	-	-	32.7	-	15–49
INDONESIA	223,040	62.1	65.9	-	63.2	52.4	-	-	15+
IRAN, ISLAMIC REPUBLIC OF	70,098	24.0	29.6	-	24.1	20.9	-	-	15–64
IRAQ	28,221	25.1	25.8	-	41.5	5.0	-	-	25–65
IRELAND	4,268	26.5	26.5	-	-	-	24.9	-	15+
ISRAEL	7,049	31.1	31.1	-	-	13.9	-	-	21+
ITALY	58,843	32.8	32.8	-	28.3	-	-	-	14+
JAMAICA	2,667	18.8	20.8	-	-	-	28.6	-	15–49
JAPAN	127,760	44.3	44.3	-	-	-	43.3	-	20+
JORDAN	5,538	61.9	62.7	-	-	-	50.5	-	18+
KAZAKHSTAN	15,308	43.2	43.2	-	52.2	38.7	-	-	18+
KENYA	36,553	23.9	27.1	-	26.2	21.2	-	-	18+
KIRIBATI	100	-	-	-	56.5	-	-	-	16+
KOREA, DEMOCRATIC PEOPLE'S REP. OF	23,708	58.6	58.6	-	59.9	-	-	-	16+
KOREA, REPUBLIC OF	48,418	53.3	53.3	-	-	-	52.8	-	20+
KUWAIT	2,599	-	-	-	34.4	-	-	-	18–60
KYRGYZSTAN	5,192	46.9	46.9	-	45.0	-	41.7	-	15+
LAO PEOPLE'S DEMOCRATIC REPUBLIC	5,759	61.1	65.0	-	65.8	59.0	-	-	18+
LATVIA	2,288	54.4	54.4	-	53.0	47.3	-	-	15–64
LEBANON	3,759	29.1	29.1	-	61.0	-	42.3	-	25–64

Female Age Standardized		Female Crude						Student Health Professionals' Smoking Prevalence (percentages)	Youth Smoking Prevalence (percentages national data)		Secondhand Smoking: Youth exposed in home (percentages)	Cigarette Consumption (annual per capita)	COUNTRY
Current Cigarette Use	Current Any Tobacco Use	Current Tobacco Use	Current Tobacco Smoking	Daily Tobacco Smoking	Current Cigarette Use	Daily Cigarette Use	Age Range		Boys	Girls			
-	-	-	10.0	-	-	-	13+	-	8.6	2.6	43.0	-	DJIBOUTI
-	-	-	-	-	-	-		-	11.8	9.6	26.4	-	DOMINICA
10.9	13.3	-	12.5	10.8	-	-	18+	-	7.3	5.8	35.0	335	DOMINICAN REPUBLIC
5.6	5.8	-	6.6	1.3	-	-	18+	-	-	-	-	234	ECUADOR
0.9	1.3	-	2.7	0.4	-	-	18+	8.0	5.9	1.4	38.0	1,082	EGYPT
-	-	3.4	-	-	-	-	12–64	-	18.4	10.9	16.1	275	EL SALVADOR
-	-	-	-	-	-	-		-	-	-	-	-	EQUATORIAL GUINEA
0.7	1.2	-	-	-	-	-		-	2.0	0.6	18.7	-	ERITREA
27.5	27.5	-	30.7	21.1	-	-	16–64	-	30.4	18.2	80.6	1,718	ESTONIA
0.5	0.9	-	0.5	0.4	-	-	18+	-	-	-	16.7	52	ETHIOPIA
5.1	5.1	-	-	3.9	-	-	15–85	-	6.7	3.1	46.5	-	FIJI
24.4	24.4	-	24.5	18.0	-	-	15–64	-	28.3	32.2	-	956	FINLAND
26.7	26.7	-	26.5	21.7	-	-	12–75	33.0	26.0	26.7	-	876	FRANCE
-	-	-	-	-	-	-		-	-	-	-	-	GABON
0.5	2.9	-	4.4	-	-	-	15+	-	-	-	-	-	GAMBIA
6.3	6.3	-	5.4	4.1	-	-	18+	-	35.5	12.9	95.0	1,040	GEORGIA
-	-	27.3	-	-	-	-	18+	52.0	32.2	33.7	-	1,125	GERMANY
0.5	0.8	-	1.2	0.4	-	-	18+	1.0	2.8	2.3	18.1	80	GHANA
39.8	39.8	-	-	-	39.0	39.6	18–89	41.0	11.3	9.0	89.8	3,017	GREECE
-	-	-	-	-	-	-		-	10.9	9.5	27.3	-	GRENADA
4.1	4.1	-	3.4	0.9	-	-	18+	-	-	-	-	325	GUATEMALA
-	-	-	8.6	-	-	-	11–72	-	-	-	-	-	GUINEA
-	-	-	-	-	-	-		-	-	-	-	-	GUINEA-BISSAU
-	-	-	-	-	-	-		-	11.0	5.4	33.7	-	GUYANA
-	-	-	4.4	-	-	-	15–49	-	14.4	12.4	26.2	-	HAITI
3.4	3.4	-	-	-	2.3	-	15–49	-	-	-	30.8	450	HONDURAS
-	-	-	-	-	-	3.5	15+	-	-	-	-	499	HONG KONG
33.9	33.9	-	31.3	27.7	-	-	18+	34.0	26.7	26.8	84.0	1,623	HUNGARY
26.6	26.6	-	23.0	19.2	-	-	15–89	-	-	-	-	-	ICELAND
1.0	3.8	3.1	-	-	1.4	-	15–49	12.0	5.9	1.8	26.5	99	INDIA
4.0	4.5	-	4.5	3.3	-	-	15+	9.0	23.9	1.9	66.8	974	INDONESIA
1.9	5.5	-	4.3	2.9	-	-	15–64	3.0	3.2	1.0	42.9	764	IRAN, ISLAMIC REPUBLIC OF
1.9	2.5	-	6.9	4.1	-	-	25–65	18.0	-	-	50.2	784	IRAQ
26.0	26.0	-	-	-	25.3	-	15+	10.0	19.5	20.5	-	1,391	IRELAND
17.9	17.9	-	-	9.1	-	-	21+	22.0	16.9	11.6	-	1,173	ISRAEL
19.2	19.2	-	16.2	-	-	-	14+	51.0	21.8	24.9	-	1,596	ITALY
7.6	9.2	-	-	-	7.7	-	15–49	-	20.6	10.9	34.4	480	JAMAICA
14.3	14.3	-	-	-	12.0	-	20+	24.0	-	-	-	2,028	JAPAN
9.8	9.8	-	-	-	8.3	-	18+	17.0	13.2	7.1	65.0	846	JORDAN
9.7	9.7	-	9.6	5.8	-	-	18+	-	12.7	6.6	72.7	1,805	KAZAKHSTAN
1.1	2.2	-	1.9	0.9	-	-	18+	-	8.7	4.7	-	167	KENYA
-	-	-	32.3	-	-	-	16+	-	-	-	-	-	KIRIBATI
-	-	-	-	-	-	-		-	-	-	-	714	KOREA, DEMOCRATIC PEOPLE'S REP. OF
5.7	5.7	-	-	-	5.8	-	20+	4.0	9.4	2.6	39.9	1,733	KOREA, REPUBLIC OF
-	-	-	1.9	-	-	-	18–60	-	17.7	4.5	-	1,509	KUWAIT
2.2	2.2	-	1.6	-	1.5	-	15+	-	7.6	4.2	64.4	1,017	KYRGYZSTAN
13.6	15.6	-	15.4	13.2	-	-	18+	-	-	-	42.9	544	LAO PEOPLE'S DEMOCRATIC REPUBLIC
24.1	24.1	-	23.7	17.8	-	-	15–64	-	36.3	30.2	-	1,890	LATVIA
7.0	7.0	-	57.1	-	30.6	-	25–64	27.0	11.8	5.6	78.9	1,837	LEBANON

101

TABLE A THE DEMOGRAPHICS OF TOBACCO

	1 Population	2 Adult Smoking Prevalence—Male (percentages)							
		Male Age Standardized		Male Crude					
COUNTRY	(thousands)	Current Cigarette Use	Current Any Tobacco Use	Current Tobacco Use	Current Tobacco Smoking	Daily Tobacco Smoking	Current Cigarette Use	Daily Cigarette Use	Age Range
LESOTHO	1,995	-	-	-	47.9	-	-	-	15+
LIBERIA	3,579	-	-	-	-	-	-	-	-
LIBYAN ARAB JAMAHIRIYA	6,039	-	-	-	-	32.0	-	-	18+
LITHUANIA	3,395	45.1	45.1	-	45.8	39.0	-	-	20-64
LUXEMBOURG	462	39.1	39.1	-	36.0	-	-	-	15+
MACEDONIA, FORMER YUGOSLAV REP.	2,036	-	-	-	-	-	-	40.0	15+
MADAGASCAR	19,159	-	-	-	-	-	-	-	-
MALAWI	13,571	19.2	23.7	-	25.5	20.6	-	-	18+
MALAYSIA	26,114	51.1	54.4	-	46.5	39.0	-	-	25-64
MALDIVES	300	39.7	44.5	37.4	-	-	27.3	-	16+
MALI	11,968	14.0	19.5	-	24.1	18.8	-	-	18+
MALTA	406	32.8	32.8	-	-	-	-	29.9	15-98
MARSHALL ISLANDS	65	-	-	-	-	-	-	-	-
MAURITANIA	3,044	16.3	22.3	-	27.4	23.2	-	-	18+
MAURITIUS	1,253	35.7	35.7	-	42.4	32.2	-	-	18+
MEXICO	104,220	36.9	36.9	-	-	-	30.4	21.6	20+
MICRONESIA, FEDERATED STATES OF	111	-	-	-	42.0	-	-	-	20-85
MOLDOVA, REPUBLIC OF	3,833	45.8	45.8	-	-	-	51.1	-	15-59
MONACO	33	-	-	-	-	-	-	-	-
MONGOLIA	2,585	45.8	45.8	-	48.4	43.1	-	-	15-64
MONTENEGRO	601	-	-	-	-	-	-	-	-
MOROCCO	30,497	26.1	29.5	-	-	30.3	-	27.4	18+
MOZAMBIQUE	20,971	20.0	22.0	38.8	-	-	-	16.7	25-64
MYANMAR	48,379	43.6	46.5	-	48.9	35.6	-	-	18+
NAMIBIA	2,047	35.9	38.6	-	28.0	22.3	-	-	18+
NAURU	14	46.1	46.1	-	49.7	45.5	-	-	15-64
NEPAL	27,641	29.3	34.8	-	-	-	30.2	-	15-49
NETHERLANDS	16,340	38.3	38.3	-	-	31.0	-	-	15+
NEW ZEALAND	4,185	29.7	29.7	-	-	-	-	21.9	15+
NICARAGUA	5,532	-	-	-	-	-	-	-	-
NIGER	13,737	-	-	-	40.6	-	-	-	15-35
NIGERIA	144,720	9.1	13.0	-	-	-	-	-	-
NIUE	1	-	-	-	-	-	37.5	-	15+
NORWAY	4,660	33.6	33.6	-	-	-	39.0	27.0	16-74
OMAN	2,546	24.1	24.7	-	13.4	-	-	-	20+
PAKISTAN	159,000	29.7	35.4	-	32.4	27.3	-	-	18+
PALAU	20	38.1	38.1	-	-	-	-	-	-
PALESTINIAN TERRITORY, OCCUPIED	3,775	-	-	-	40.7	-	-	-	Adult
PANAMA	3,288	-	-	-	52.1	-	-	-	15-75
PAPUA NEW GUINEA	6,202	-	-	-	46.0	-	-	-	15+
PARAGUAY	6,016	32.6	33.0	-	41.6	23.5	-	-	18+
PERU	27,589	-	-	-	42.6	-	-	-	12-64
PHILIPPINES	86,264	38.9	42.0	-	57.5	40.3	-	-	18+
POLAND	38,129	43.9	43.9	-	-	-	-	38.0	15+
PORTUGAL	10,589	40.6	40.6	-	-	-	35.0	-	18+
QATAR	821	-	-	-	37.0	-	-	-	Adult
ROMANIA	21,590	40.6	40.6	-	33.0	-	-	-	15-59
RUSSIAN FEDERATION	142,500	70.1	70.1	-	-	-	-	60.4	18+
RWANDA	9,464	-	-	-	-	-	-	-	-

Female Age Standardized		Female Crude						Student Health Professionals' Smoking Prevalence	Youth Smoking Prevalence		Secondhand Smoking: Youth exposed in home	Cigarette Consumption	
Current Cigarette Use	Current Any Tobacco Use	Current Tobacco Use	Current Tobacco Smoking	Daily Tobacco Smoking	Current Cigarette Use	Daily Cigarette Use	Age Range	(percentages)	(percentages national data) Boys	Girls	(percentages)	(annual per capita)	COUNTRY
-	-	-	34.2	-	-	-	15+	-	16.6	4.8	-	-	LESOTHO
-	-	-	-	-	-	-	-	-	-	-	-	-	LIBERIA
-	-	-	-	1.5	-	-	18+	-	7.7	0.9	40.3	860	LIBYAN ARAB JAMAHIRIYA
20.8	20.8	-	20.3	14.0	-	-	20-64	28.0	33.8	25.9	45.0	920	LITHUANIA
30.3	30.3	-	26.0	-	-	-	15+	-	-	-	-	-	LUXEMBOURG
-	-	-	-	-	-	32.0	15+	-	8.5	6.8	91.9	2,336	MACEDONIA, FORMER YUGOSLAV REP.
-	-	-	-	-	-	-	-	-	-	-	-	276	MADAGASCAR
2.3	6.2	-	6.1	5.1	-	-	18+	-	3.8	2.2	10.8	-	MALAWI
2.5	2.8	-	3.0	2.1	-	-	25-64	2.0	36.3	4.2	59.0	646	MALAYSIA
8.9	11.6	15.6	-	-	2.2	-	16+	-	9.0	3.1	50.2	-	MALDIVES
0.7	2.8	-	2.3	1.6	-	-	18+	-	-	-	-	-	MALI
24.5	24.5	-	-	-	-	17.6	15-98	-	16.9	17.4	-	1,287	MALTA
-	-	-	-	-	-	-	-	-	-	-	-	-	MARSHALL ISLANDS
0.8	3.7	-	4.2	3.2	-	-	18+	-	20.3	18.3	43.8	-	MAURITANIA
1.1	1.1	-	2.9	1.1	-	-	18+	-	19.8	7.7	42.7	846	MAURITIUS
12.4	12.4	-	-	-	9.5	6.5	20+	-	-	-	46.9	470	MEXICO
-	-	-	-	-	-	-	-	-	36.9	19.8	60.6	-	MICRONESIA, FEDERATED STATES OF
5.8	5.8	-	-	-	7.1	-	15-49	-	23.0	6.0	62.3	2,239	MOLDOVA, REPUBLIC OF
-	-	-	-	-	-	-	-	-	-	-	-	-	MONACO
6.5	6.5	-	5.5	4.1	-	-	15-64	-	14.4	4.0	64.2	-	MONGOLIA
-	-	-	-	-	-	-	-	-	6.0	5.0	96.2	-	MONTENEGRO
0.2	0.3	-	-	0.2	-	0.2	18+	-	4.3	2.1	30.0	430	MOROCCO
1.6	3.4	15.0	-	-	-	1.9	25-64	-	-	-	-	213	MOZAMBIQUE
11.7	13.6	-	13.7	10.4	-	-	18+	13.0	19.0	3.2	-	209	MYANMAR
9.2	10.9	-	12.4	9.4	-	-	18+	-	21.9	16.1	41.5	-	NAMIBIA
52.4	52.4	-	56.0	50.8	-	-	15-64	-	-	-	-	-	NAURU
26.2	26.4	-	-	-	15.2	-	15-49	-	-	-	84.7	274	NEPAL
30.3	30.3	-	25.0	-	-	-	15+	24.0	22.5	24.3	-	888	NETHERLANDS
27.5	27.5	-	-	-	-	19.5	15+	-	13.0	23.9	-	565	NEW ZEALAND
-	-	-	5.3	-	-	-	15-49	-	-	-	41.5	386	NICARAGUA
-	-	-	11.3	-	-	-	15-35	-	11.7	1.1	33.9	-	NIGER
0.2	1.2	-	1.0	-	0.5	-	15-49	-	9.7	5.7	-	103	NIGERIA
-	-	-	-	-	14.5	-	15+	-	-	-	-	-	NIUE
30.4	30.4	-	-	-	35.0	24.0	16-74	-	15.4	19.9	-	493	NORWAY
0.3	1.3	-	0.5	-	-	-	20+	-	3.5	1.2	21.8	-	OMAN
2.8	6.6	-	5.7	4.4	-	-	18+	14.0	-	-	29.6	391	PAKISTAN
9.7	9.7	-	-	-	-	-	-	-	31.0	22.6	-	-	PALAU
-	-	-	3.2	-	-	-	Adult	-	-	-	-	-	PALESTINIAN TERRITORY, OCCUPIED
-	-	-	19.5	-	-	-	15-75	-	14.7	11.1	-	291	PANAMA
-	-	-	28.0	-	-	-	15+	-	52.1	35.8	76.0	-	PAPUA NEW GUINEA
13.9	14.8	-	13.3	6.5	-	-	18+	-	-	-	42.5	968	PARAGUAY
-	-	-	22.5	-	-	-	12-64	26.0	-	-	28.7	129	PERU
8.5	9.8	-	12.3	7.1	-	-	18+	22.0	23.4	11.8	56.4	1,073	PHILIPPINES
27.2	27.2	-	-	-	-	25.6	15+	39.0	19.6	17.1	87.9	1,810	POLAND
31.0	31.0	-	-	-	17.6	-	18+	18.0	17.6	26.2	-	1,318	PORTUGAL
-	-	-	0.5	-	-	-	Adult	-	13.4	2.3	32.0	-	QATAR
24.5	24.5	-	27.1	-	-	-	15-59	40.0	21.5	14.3	89.4	1,480	ROMANIA
26.5	26.5	-	-	-	-	15.5	18+	39.0	26.9	23.9	75.2	2,319	RUSSIAN FEDERATION
-	-	8.3	-	-	-	-	15-49	-	-	-	-	-	RWANDA

TABLE A THE DEMOGRAPHICS OF TOBACCO

	1	2							
	Population	Adult Smoking Prevalence—Male (percentages)							
COUNTRY		Male Age Standardized		Male Crude					
	(thousands)	Current Cigarette Use	Current Any Tobacco Use	Current Tobacco Use	Current Tobacco Smoking	Daily Tobacco Smoking	Current Cigarette Use	Daily Cigarette Use	Age Range
SAINT KITTS AND NEVIS	48	-	-	-	-	-	-	-	-
SAINT LUCIA	166	25.4	28.9	-	-	-	37.3	-	25+
SAINT VINCENT AND GRENADINES	120	18.7	-	-	-	-	26.4	17.4	19+
SAMOA	185	58.3	58.3	-	-	-	60.0	-	29+
SAN MARINO	29	-	-	-	28.0	-	-	-	14+
SAO TOME AND PRINCIPE	155	23.2	23.2	-	-	-	-	28.8	14+
SAUDI ARABIA	23,679	25.1	25.6	-	-	37.6	-	-	15+
SENEGAL	12,072	14.4	19.8	-	22.2	19.8	-	-	18+
SERBIA AND MONTENEGRO	7,439	43.8	42.3	-	-	-	-	36.0	15+
SEYCHELLES	85	30.8	35.2	-	-	-	-	30.8	25-64
SIERRA LEONE	5,743	-	-	-	-	-	32.3	-	15+
SINGAPORE	4,484	25.5	-	-	-	-	24.9	21.8	18-69
SLOVAKIA	5,390	41.6	41.6	-	40.8	32.8	-	-	18+
SLOVENIA	2,007	31.8	31.8	-	28.3	25.3	-	-	18+
SOLOMON ISLANDS	484	-	-	-	-	-	-	-	-
SOMALIA	8,445	-	-	-	-	-	-	-	-
SOUTH AFRICA	47,391	25.0	27.5	-	36.0	27.1	-	-	18+
SPAIN	44,121	36.4	36.4	-	40.0	34.1	-	-	18+
SRI LANKA	19,886	24.5	30.2	-	39.0	24.5	-	-	18+
SUDAN	37,707	-	-	-	23.5	-	-	-	adult
SURINAME	455	-	-	-	-	-	-	-	-
SWAZILAND	1,138	13.3	14.6	-	13.8	9.9	-	-	18+
SWEDEN	9,084	19.6	19.6	-	-	16.5	-	-	18-64
SWITZERLAND	7,491	30.7	30.7	-	-	-	35.0	24.0	15-65
SYRIAN ARAB REPUBLIC	19,408	42.6	44.0	-	51.0	47.0	-	-	15+
TAJIKISTAN	6,640	-	-	-	-	-	-	-	-
TANZANIA, UNITED REPUBLIC OF	39,459	20.5	24.8	-	-	-	-	23.0	25-64
THAILAND	63,444	37.1	39.8	-	-	-	40.2	-	11+
TIMOR-LESTE	1,029	25.7	-	37.0	-	-	30.5	-	NA
TOGO	6,410	-	-	-	-	-	-	-	-
TONGA	100	61.8	61.8	-	-	-	52.9	-	15+
TRINIDAD AND TOBAGO	1,328	32.2	36.4	-	29.8	-	-	-	15+
TUNISIA	10,128	46.5	51.0	-	52.1	50.3	-	-	18+
TURKEY	72,975	51.6	51.6	-	52.0	49.9	-	-	18+
TURKMENISTAN	4,900	-	-	-	27.0	-	-	-	18+
TUVALU	12	-	-	-	51.0	-	-	-	20+
UGANDA	29,899	18.4	20.9	-	25.2	-	-	-	15-54
UKRAINE	46,788	63.8	63.8	-	66.8	62.3	-	-	15+
UNITED ARAB EMIRATES	4,249	25.5	26.1	-	28.1	17.6	-	-	18+
UNITED KINGDOM *	60,550	-	-	-	22	-	22	-	16+
UNITED STATES OF AMERICA	299,400	-	-	-	-	-	23.9	-	18+
URUGUAY	3,315	37.1	37.1	-	38.8	33.8	-	-	18+
UZBEKISTAN	26,540	24.2	24.2	-	-	-	22.6	-	15-59
VANUATU	221	49.1	49.1	-	49.1	-	-	37.4	20+
VENEZUELA	27,021	32.5	32.5	-	22.6	20.9	-	-	15+
VIETNAM	84,108	42.9	45.7	-	49.4	34.8	-	-	18+
YEMEN	21,732	-	-	-	77.0	-	-	-	adult
ZAMBIA	11,696	18.0	21.7	-	22.7	15.3	-	-	18+
ZIMBABWE	13,228	21.2	25.5	-	-	33.4	-	26.7	18+

* does not include data from Northern Ireland

Female Age Standardized		Female Crude						Student Health Professionals' Smoking Prevalence	Youth Smoking Prevalence (percentages national data)		Secondhand Smoking: Youth exposed in home	Cigarette Consumption	COUNTRY
Current Cigarette Use	Current Any Tobacco Use	Current Tobacco Use	Current Tobacco Smoking	Daily Tobacco Smoking	Current Cigarette Use	Daily Cigarette Use	Age Range	(percentages)	Boys	Girls	(percentages)	(annual per capita)	
-	-	-	-	-	-	-	-	-	7.0	1.9	-	-	SAINT KITTS AND NEVIS
9.2	12.1	-	-	-	5.6	-	25+	-	17.0	9.6	25.3	-	SAINT LUCIA
5.3	-	-	-	-	3.5	1.9	19+	-	14.8	9.5	-	-	SAINT VINCENT AND GRENADINES
23.4	23.4	-	-	-	24.0	-	29+	-	16.0	12.7	58.9	-	SAMOA
-	-	-	17.0	-	-	-	14+	-	-	-	-	-	SAN MARINO
10.6	10.6	-	-	-	-	14.3	14+	-	-	-	-	-	SAO TOME AND PRINCIPE
3.4	3.6	-	-	6.0	-	-	15+	12.0	10.2	2.6	-	648	SAUDI ARABIA
0.6	1.5	-	1.7	1.0	-	-	18+	-	12.1	2.7	-	380	SENEGAL
43.8	42.3	-	-	-	-	36.0	15+	35.0 (Serbia only)	12.2	13.1	97.4 (Serbia only)	-	SERBIA AND MONTENEGRO
3.0	7.0	-	-	-	-	3.9	25-64	-	29.9	23.9	-	-	SEYCHELLES
4.1	-	-	-	-	10.3	-	15+	-	-	-	-	-	SIERRA LEONE
4.9	-	-	-	-	4.1	3.5	18-69	-	10.5	7.5	-	406	SINGAPORE
20.1	20.1	-	23.0	14.3	-	-	18+	30.0	28.1	24.3	79.5	1,430	SLOVAKIA
21.1	21.1	-	18.4	16.8	-	-	18	-	21.4	23.9	68.1	2,537	SLOVENIA
-	-	-	23.0	-	-	-	15+	-	-	-	-	-	SOLOMON ISLANDS
-	-	-	-	-	-	-	-	-	-	-	51.8	-	SOMALIA
7.8	9.1	-	10.2	8.2	-	-	18+	-	21.0	10.6	-	511	SOUTH AFRICA
30.9	30.9	-	26.8	23.7	-	-	18+	37.0	23.6	32.3	-	2,225	SPAIN
0.4	2.6	-	2.6	1.6	-	-	18+	4.0	3.0	1.3	51.3	205	SRI LANKA
-	-	-	1.5	-	-	-	Adult	-	10.2	2.1	28.4	75	SUDAN
-	-	-	-	-	-	-	-	-	9.3	4.7	50.5	-	SURINAME
2.8	3.2	-	3.3	2.1	-	-	18+	-	8.9	3.2	27.1	-	SWAZILAND
24.5	24.5	-	-	18.8	-	-	18-64	-	5.5	13.7	-	751	SWEDEN
22.2	22.2	-	-	-	26.0	19.0	15-65	-	12.9	13.0	-	1,698	SWITZERLAND
-	-	-	10.0	8.0	-	-	15+	17.0	8.1	3.1	-	1,067	SYRIAN ARAB REPUBLIC
-	-	-	-	-	-	-	-	-	1.5	0.5	54.5	-	TAJIKISTAN
1.7	4.3	-	-	-	-	1.3	25-64	-	-	-	30.6	108	TANZANIA, UNITED REPUBLIC OF
3.0	3.4	-	-	-	2.4	-	11+	1.0	17.4	4.8	47.8	634	THAILAND
0.9	-	6.1	-	-	1.3	-	NA	-	50.6	17.3	65.1	-	TIMOR-LESTE
-	-	-	-	-	-	-	-	-	9.1	1.7	20.2	306	TOGO
15.8	15.8	-	-	-	10.5	-	15+	-	-	-	-	-	TONGA
5.7	7.6	-	5.1	-	-	-	15+	-	14.7	10.3	40.7	1,337	TRINIDAD AND TOBAGO
1.0	1.9	-	2.0	1.9	-	-	18+	11.0	15.1	1.6	-	1,532	TUNISIA
19.2	19.2	-	17.3	15.6	-	-	18+	33.0	9.4	3.5	89.0	1,499	TURKEY
-	-	-	1.0	-	-	-	18+	-	-	-	-	496	TURKMENISTAN
-	-	-	31.0	-	-	-	20+	-	33.2	22.1	74.8	-	TUVALU
1.5	3.2	-	3.3	-	-	-	15-49	3.0	6.6	4.0	-	-	UGANDA
22.7	22.7	-	19.9	16.7	-	-	15+	-	27.6	20.6	70.1	2,526	UKRAINE
1.6	2.6	-	2.4	1.4	-	-	18+	-	12.1	3.6	26.5	1,092	UNITED ARAB EMIRATES
-	-	-	20	-	20	-	16+	7.0	20.3	27.4	-	790	UNITED KINGDOM *
-	-	27.3	-	-	18	-	18+	4.0	12.1	13.9	41.1	1,196	UNITED STATES OF AMERICA
28.0	28.0	-	28.4	23.4	-	-	18+	-	16.4	22.9	51.1	793	URUGUAY
1.2	1.2	-	-	-	0.9	-	15-49	-	-	-	-	317	UZBEKISTAN
8.1	8.1	-	5.0	-	-	3.2	20+	-	28.2	11.4	74.0	-	VANUATU
27.0	27.0	-	13.6	13.0	-	-	15+	-	6.0	8.4	44.3	622	VENEZUELA
2.2	2.5	-	2.3	1.8	-	-	18+	11.0	-	-	55.3	887	VIETNAM
-	-	-	29.0	-	-	-	adult	-	6.5	3.0	44.0	317	YEMEN
2.1	5.0	-	5.7	3.4	-	-	18+	-	-	-	-	71	ZAMBIA
2.0	4.4	-	-	5.0	-	1.4	18+	-	-	-	27.4	86	ZIMBABWE

* does not include data from Northern Ireland 105

TABLE B THE BUSINESS OF TOBACCO

COUNTRY	1 Growing Tobacco			2 Tobacco Trade			
	Tobacco Harvest Area (hectares, 2004-2007)	Agricultural Land under Tobacco (percent of total, 2005)	Tobacco Produced (metric tons, 2006)	Cigarette Exports (millions, 2002-2007)	Cigarette Imports (millions, 2004-2007)	Tobacco Leaf Exports (metric tons, 2006)	Tobacco Leaf Imports (metric tons, 2006)
AFGHANISTAN	–	–	–	–	–	–	–
ALBANIA	1,200	0.1336	2,000	1	4,220	1,217	10
ALGERIA	5,500	0.0119	6,889	4	1,266	0	18,592
ANDORRA	–	–	–	1	332	334	–
ANGOLA	3,500	–	3,300	–	–	–	–
ANTIGUA AND BARBUDA	–	–	–	–	–	–	–
ARGENTINA	92,000	–	165,000	703	4	100,498	3,728
ARMENIA	500	0.0151	200	500	3,250	77	3,410
AUSTRALIA	1,417	0.0003	4,000	6,865	2,960	1,386	19,921
AUSTRIA	200	0.0030	304	31,791	8,344	458	19,757
AZERBAIJAN	1,191	0.0584	4,845	638	13,366	4,455	3,869
BAHAMAS	–	–	–	0	0	0	43
BAHRAIN	–	–	–	57	1,771	–	61
BANGLADESH	30,000	0.3323	38,000	1,055	478	–	–
BARBADOS	–	–	–	0	138	–	2
BELARUS	820	0.0090	1,600	1,200	3,337	134	9,061
BELGIUM	71	0.0234	209	857	22,752	45,520	62,033
BELIZE	–	–	–	3	260	–	36
BENIN	1,350	0.0392	1,000	1,544	301	–	–
BHUTAN	110	0.0186	–	–	–	–	–
BOLIVIA	850	0.0023	1,170	83	282	–	285
BOSNIA AND HERZEGOVINA	2,321	0.1352	3,916	328	6,675	846	1,932
BOTSWANA	–	–	–	–	675	–	128
BRAZIL	461,482	0.1873	900,381	5,197	115	566,027	10,119
BRUNEI DARUSSALAM	–	–	–	–	–	–	–
BULGARIA	29,900	0.7762	41,956	2,446	193	38,661	11,112
BURKINA FASO	1,050	0.0101	500	1,075	176	–	–
BURUNDI	970	0.0417	770	169	353	522	135
CAMBODIA	8,500	0.1527	14,231	197	17,780	–	–
CAMEROON	3,400	0.0371	4,500	3	687	512	131
CANADA	16,500	0.0237	43,000	8,071	17,392	14,381	5,591
CAPE VERDE	–	–	–	9	51	–	28
CENTRAL AFRICAN REPUBLIC	600	0.0115	475	–	–	–	–
CHAD	150	0.0003	180	–	–	–	–
CHILE	3,000	0.0203	8,349	5,758	123	274	4,905
CHINA	1,401,200	0.2453	2,746,193	24,513	3,836	147,028	82,390
COLOMBIA	18,000	0.0413	35,000	6,963	3,387	6,873	1,373
COMOROS	–	–	–	–	54	–	–
CONGO	700	0.0066	300	–	–	–	–
CONGO, DEMOCRATIC REPUBLIC OF THE	8,200	0.0373	4,000	–	–	–	–
COOK ISLANDS	–	–	–	–	11	–	–
COSTA RICA	75	0.0019	136	11	39	149	1,037
COTE D'IVOIRE	20,000	0.0985	10,200	883	747	84	4,090
CROATIA	5,300	0.1904	10,851	7,345	1,233	5,897	4,722
CUBA	27,500	0.3079	29,700	738	65	2,770	176
CYPRUS	100	–	360	2,722	3,725	0	1
CZECH REPUBLIC	–	–	–	9,477	17,064	3,039	16,342
DENMARK	–	–	–	5,066	4,632	920	15,745

Cigarettes Manufactured (millions, 2007 or latest)	Marlboro or Equivalent (USD per pack)	Local Brand (USD per pack)	as a proportion of retail price	Signed	Ratified or acceded	on the Legacy Website 2008	Country Income Classification (World Bank, July 2008)	COUNTRY
3 Manufacturing	4 Price		5 Tax	6 WHO FCTC		7 Tobacco Industry Documents		
–	$0.40	$0.40	–	29-Jun-04	–	3,175	Low	AFGHANISTAN
4	$1.83	$1.29	58.30%	29-Jun-04	26-Apr-06	3,403	Lower middle	ALBANIA
17,500	$2.88	$0.93	63.53%	20-Jun-03	30-Jun-06	5,227	Lower middle	ALGERIA
–	–	–	–	–	–	2,810	High	ANDORRA
3,800	$1.90	$0.50	10.00%	29-Jun-04	20-Sep-07	5,296	Lower middle	ANGOLA
–	–	–	–	28-Jun-04	5-Jun-06	3,484	High	ANTIGUA AND BARBUDA
38,000	$1.14	$0.98	68.10%	25-Sep-03	–	65,479	Upper middle	ARGENTINA
2,825	$1.92	$0.50	60.67%	–	29-Nov-04	2,571	Lower middle	ARMENIA
23,300	$7.81	$7.41	62.09%	5-Dec-03	27-Oct-04	170,044	High	AUSTRALIA
40,810	$5.47	$5.75	74.90%	28-Aug-03	15-Sep-05	50,468	High	AUSTRIA
4,620	$1.33	$0.65	–	–	1-Nov-05	2,870	Lower middle	AZERBAIJAN
–	–	–	–	29-Jun-04	–	5,616	High	BAHAMAS
–	$1.45	–	68.00%	–	20-Mar-07	9,509	High	BAHRAIN
22,524	$1.16	$0.58	65.00%	16-Jun-03	14-Jun-04	22,775	Low	BANGLADESH
270	$2.51	$2.51	24.39%	28-Jun-04	3-Nov-05	13,958	High	BARBADOS
15,650	$0.50	$0.50	29.90%	17-Jun-04	8-Sep-05	3,423	Upper middle	BELARUS
9,500	$5.89	$5.81	77.43%	22-Jan-04	1-Nov-05	91,832	High	BELGIUM
100	$2.55	$2.55	–	26-Sep-03	15-Dec-05	2,080	Upper middle	BELIZE
–	$0.75	$0.75	17.25%	18-Jun-04	3-Nov-05	3,594	Low	BENIN
–	–	–	–	9-Dec-03	23-Aug-04	861	Lower middle	BHUTAN
1,350	$1.30	$0.75	43.00%	27-Feb-04	15-Sep-05	6,953	Lower middle	BOLIVIA
4,537	$2.41	$2.41	67.70%	–	–	3,450	Lower middle	BOSNIA AND HERZEGOVINA
–	–	–	39.09%	16-Jun-03	31-Jan-05	1,566	Upper middle	BOTSWANA
111,450	$1.59	$1.44	68.20%	16-Jun-03	3-Nov-05	127,215	Upper middle	BRAZIL
–	$2.30	$1.64	–	3-Jun-04	3-Jun-04	3,962	High	BRUNEI DARUSSALAM
17,500	$2.54	$1.31	81.56%	22-Dec-03	7-Nov-05	23,118	Upper middle	BULGARIA
–	$0.65	$0.65	27.25%	22-Dec-03	31-Jul-06	2,393	Low	BURKINA FASO
1,360	$0.65	$0.65	55.53%	16-Jun-03	22-Nov-05	1,443	Low	BURUNDI
4,150	$1.00	$0.85	19.80%	25-May-04	15-Nov-05	6,573	Low	CAMBODIA
1,689	$1.44	$0.78	38.70%	13-May-04	3-Feb-06	11,675	Lower middle	CAMEROON
25,146	$8.05	$8.08	69.27%	15-Jul-03	26-Nov-04	262,312	High	CANADA
40	–	–	20.04%	17-Feb-04	4-Oct-05	989	Lower middle	CAPE VERDE
–	–	–	31.97%	29-Dec-03	7-Nov-05	7,624	Low	CENTRAL AFRICAN REPUBLIC
–	$0.60	$0.60	33.25%	22-Jun-04	30-Jan-06	17,296	Low	CHAD
18,200	$2.88	$2.17	77.25%	25-Sep-03	13-Jun-05	49,567	Upper middle	CHILE
2,158,200	$2.04	$1.70	35.00%–40.00%	10-Nov-03	11-Oct-05	114,342	Lower middle	CHINA
25,000	$1.14	$0.83	49.79%	–	10-Apr-08	23,487	Lower middle	COLOMBIA
–	–	–	80.09%	27-Feb-04	24-Jan-06	552	Low	COMOROS
1,040	$0.65	$0.65	31.25%	23-Mar-04	6-Feb-07	15,357	Lower middle	CONGO
6,500	$0.38	$0.38	38.50%	28-Jun-04	28-Oct-05	9,988	Low	CONGO, DEMOCRATIC REPUBLIC OF THE
–	–	–	–	14-May-04	14-May-04	2,895	–	COOK ISLANDS
854	$1.35	$1.21	56.50%	3-Jul-03	21-Aug-08	27,978	Upper middle	COSTA RICA
3,500	$2.52	$1.68	50.25%	24-Jul-03	–	233	Low	COTE D'IVOIRE
14,457	$3.28	$3.24	67.10%	2-Jun-04	14-Jul-08	4,360	Upper middle	CROATIA
13,200	$3.00	$1.03	22.00%	29-Jun-04	–	23,471	Upper middle	CUBA
1,750	$4.67	$4.14	72.08%	24-May-04	26-Oct-05	23,310	High	CYPRUS
17,825	$3.44	$3.56	80.43%	16-Jun-03	–	14,586	High	CZECH REPUBLIC
11,849	$5.91	$5.91	73.40%	16-Jun-03	16-Dec-04	62,935	High	DENMARK

TABLE B THE BUSINESS OF TOBACCO

COUNTRY	1 Growing Tobacco		2 Tobacco Trade				
	Tobacco Harvest Area (hectares, 2004-2007)	Agricultural Land under Tobacco (percent of total, 2005)	Tobacco Produced (metric tons, 2006)	Cigarette Exports (millions, 2002-2007)	Cigarette Imports (millions, 2004-2007)	Tobacco Leaf Exports (metric tons, 2006)	Tobacco Leaf Imports (metric tons, 2006)
DJIBOUTI	–	–	–	–	–	–	–
DOMINICA	–	–	–	4	6	–	0
DOMINICAN REPUBLIC	9,000	0.2485	12,000	–	–	–	–
ECUADOR	4,100	0.0530	7,800	2	122	3,025	524
EGYPT	–	–	–	–	–	30	67,873
EL SALVADOR	600	–	1,100	1	887	–	412
EQUATORIAL GUINEA	–	–	–	–	–	–	–
ERITREA	–	–	–	–	–	–	–
ESTONIA	–	–	–	11	3,511	–	0
ETHIOPIA	4,500	0.0133	3,000	–	300	–	1,486
FIJI	500	–	310	13	52	0	75
FINLAND	–	–	–	139	6,669	–	25
FRANCE	7,000	0.0283	18,880	29,166	118,528	33,050	86,005
GABON	–	–	–	638	380	70	2,059
GAMBIA	–	–	–	–	–	–	10
GEORGIA	720	0.0166	1,371	12	1,662	1	1,745
GERMANY	4,500	0.0262	11,000	171,774	29,886	67,619	195,111
GHANA	5,750	–	2,500	27	118	190	338
GREECE	17,400	0.6504	37,252	18,500	12,575	86,402	34,016
GRENADA	–	–	–	–	–	–	–
GUATEMALA	9,500	0.1985	21,500	1,736	775	4,476	1,218
GUINEA	2,100	0.0159	1,800	83	–	–	–
GUINEA-BISSAU	–	–	–	–	–	–	–
GUYANA	100	0.0057	90	12	118	549	108
HAITI	450	0.0264	500	–	–	–	–
HONDURAS	4,200	0.1417	6,180	1,887	742	1,925	6,459
HONG KONG SAR, CHINA	–	–	–	58,424	26,938	580	12,873
HUNGARY	6,000	0.1117	9,145	2,547	10,215	2,593	3,543
ICELAND	–	–	–	–	379	–	–
INDIA	380,000	0.2034	552,200	2,240	683	158,254	1,273
INDONESIA	215,000	0.3033	177,895	–	–	51,997	48,287
IRAN, ISLAMIC REPUBLIC OF	20,000	0.4147	21,000	57	954	1,911	408
IRAQ	1,700	0.0040	2,300	–	–	30	–
IRELAND	–	–	–	7	3,728	1	6,021
ISRAEL	0	0.0000	0	33	6,178	–	2,481
ITALY	35,000	–	110,000	95	77,914	94,298	11,748
JAMAICA	1,200	–	1,800	38	1,325	0	1
JAPAN	19,000	0.4145	38,000	17,460	98,767	7,378	49,761
JORDAN	2,900	0.2866	2,100	–	–	91	3,664
KAZAKHSTAN	5,000	0.0037	13,500	3,097	2,461	5,816	16,091
KENYA	15,000	–	20,000	11,505	60	20,058	12,415
KIRIBATI	–	–	–	–	91	–	–
KOREA, DEM. PEOPLE'S REPUBLIC OF	45,000	1.5082	65,000	–	–	–	–
KOREA, REPUBLIC OF	15,000	–	34,000	48,063	481	4,093	39,266
KUWAIT	–	–	–	–	–	–	–
KYRGYZSTAN	5,800	0.0511	13,400	126	4,659	7,201	917
LAO PEOPLE'S DEMOCRATIC REPUBLIC	4,800	0.2736	–	–	–	–	–
LATVIA	–	–	–	8,854	7,031	42	2,025
LEBANON	9,000	2.3196	9,000	21	6,832	–	–

3 Manufacturing		4 Price		5 Tax	6 WHO FCTC		7 Tobacco Industry Documents		COUNTRY
Cigarettes Manufactured	Marlboro or Equivalent	Local Brand	as a proportion of retail price		Signed	Ratified or acceded	on the Legacy Website	Country Income Classification	
(millions, 2007 or latest)	(USD per pack)	(USD per pack)					2008	(World Bank, July 2008)	
-	-	-	29.00%		13-May-04	31-Jul-05	1,986	Lower middle	DJIBOUTI
-	-	-	32.04%		29-Jun-04	24-Jul-06	3,043	Upper middle	DOMINICA
2,940	$0.61	$0.50	59.79%		-	-	10,319	Lower middle	DOMINICAN REPUBLIC
2,980	$1.50	$1.48	57.71%		22-Mar-04	25-Jul-06	14,898	Lower middle	ECUADOR
80,900	$1.33	$1.28	58.00%		17-Jun-03	25-Feb-05	22,798	Lower middle	EGYPT
1,107	$1.20	$1.14	44.50%		18-Mar-04	-	18,721	Lower middle	EL SALVADOR
-	-	-	32.04%		-	17-Sep-05	607	High	EQUATORIAL GUINEA
-	-	-	50.85%		-	-	754	Low	ERITREA
1,600	$2.22	$1.95	91.50%		8-Jun-04	27-Jul-05	4,232	High	ESTONIA
3,400	$1.55	$0.42	45.04%		25-Feb-04	-	4,001	Low	ETHIOPIA
700	$3.01	$3.01	-		3-Oct-03	3-Oct-03	6,833	Upper middle	FIJI
403	$5.89	$5.75	75.07%		16-Jun-03	24-Jan-05	84,592	High	FINLAND
25,033	$7.26	$6.92	80.39%		16-Jun-03	19-Oct-04	169,804	High	FRANCE
-	-	-	45.25%		22-Aug-03	-	2,573	Upper middle	GABON
-	-	-	-		16-Jun-03	18-Sep-07	2,717	Low	GAMBIA
3,000	$1.50	$1.03	39.20%		20-Feb-04	14-Feb-06	10,460	Lower middle	GEORGIA
216,042	$6.38	$6.18	75.77%		24-Oct-03	16-Dec-04	261,058	High	GERMANY
1,500	$1.00	$0.55	67.50%		20-Jun-03	29-Nov-04	17,915	Low	GHANA
32,538	$3.77	$3.42	73.47%		16-Jun-03	27-Jan-06	55,619	High	GREECE
-	-	-	-		29-Jun-04	14-Aug-07	1,967	Upper middle	GRENADA
4,300	$1.89	$1.78	57.71%		25-Sep-03	16-Nov-05	29,890	Lower middle	GUATEMALA
85	$0.60	$0.60	28.25%		1-Apr-04	7-Nov-07	51,927	Low	GUINEA
-	-	-	-		-	7-Nov-08	814	Low	GUINEA-BISSAU
650	$0.85	$0.85	45.79%		-	15-Sep-05	9,818	Lower middle	GUYANA
880	$0.55	$0.55	-		23-Jul-03	-	4,563	Low	HAITI
6,852	$1.20	$0.90	29.71%		18-Jun-04	16-Feb-05	19,391	Lower middle	HONDURAS
17,481	$3.72	$4.15	-		-	-	119,511	High	HONG KONG
8,132	$3.06	$3.04	73.93%		16-Jun-03	7-Apr-04	34,634	High	HUNGARY
-	$8.03	$8.75	-		16-Jun-03	14-Jun-04	10,808	High	ICELAND
98,000	$1.97	$1.57	69.11%		10-Sep-03	5-Feb-04	98,503	Lower middle	INDIA
230,300	$0.90	$1.24	37.00%		-	-	49,038	Lower middle	INDONESIA
24,600	$1.82	$0.48	10.00%		16-Jun-03	6-Nov-05	25,462	Lower middle	IRAN, ISLAMIC REPUBLIC OF
5,000	$1.50	$1.00	-		29-Jun-04	17-Mar-08	7,839	Lower middle	IRAQ
3,683	$9.59	$9.59	78.38%		16-Sep-03	7-Nov-05	60,362	High	IRELAND
1,686	$4.48	$3.23	82.42%		20-Jun-03	24-Aug-05	48,035	High	ISRAEL
18,248	$5.62	$4.66	75.17%		16-Jun-03	2-Jul-08	101,416	High	ITALY
940	$4.66	$3.47	45.16%		24-Sep-03	7-Jul-05	16,422	Upper middle	JAMAICA
185,900	$2.82	$2.64	63.00%		9-Mar-04	8-Jun-04	232,096	High	JAPAN
14,993	$2.11	$7.06	51.79%		28-May-04	19-Aug-04	39,014	Lower middle	JORDAN
30,834	$1.22	$0.53	26.00%		21-Jun-04	22-Jan-07	6,028	Upper middle	KAZAKHSTAN
10,000	$1.94	$1.34	41.79%		25-Jun-04	25-Jun-04	34,027	Low	KENYA
-	-	-	-		27-Apr-04	15-Sep-05	459	Lower middle	KIRIBATI
15,500	$2.66	$0.71	-		17-Jun-03	27-Apr-05	23,560	Low	KOREA, DEM. PEOPLE'S REPUBLIC OF
126,000	$2.48	$2.15	63.09%		21-Jul-03	16-May-05	27,059	High	KOREA, REPUBLIC OF
-	$1.68	$3.00	32.00%		16-Jun-03	12-May-06	15,450	High	KUWAIT
3,086	$0.83	$0.83	26.00%		18-Feb-04	25-May-06	2,248	Low	KYRGYZSTAN
2,575	$1.18	$0.46	45.04%		29-Jun-04	6-Sep-06	5,236	Low	LAO PEOPLE'S DEMOCRATIC REPUBLIC
2,776	$0.80	$1.35	89.84%		10-May-04	10-Feb-05	3,990	Upper middle	LATVIA
555	$1.44	$0.50	57.09%		4-Mar-04	7-Dec-05	17,899	Upper middle	LEBANON

TABLE B THE BUSINESS OF TOBACCO

COUNTRY	1 Growing Tobacco		2 Tobacco Trade				
	Tobacco Harvest Area (hectares, 2004–2007)	Agricultural Land under Tobacco (percent of total, 2005)	Tobacco Produced (metric tons, 2006)	Cigarette Exports (millions, 2002–2007)	Cigarette Imports (millions, 2004–2007)	Tobacco Leaf Exports (metric tons, 2006)	Tobacco Leaf Imports (metric tons, 2006)
LESOTHO	–	–	–	–	–	–	–
LIBERIA	–	–	–	–	–	–	–
LIBYAN ARAB JAMAHIRIYA	700	0.0045	1,500	–	–	–	–
LITHUANIA	–	–	–	11,679	4,586	4	9,666
LUXEMBOURG	–	–	–	5,087	3,653	943	9,751
MACEDONIA, FORMER YUGOSLAV REP. OF	1,800	1.4886	25,036	1,933	512	29,408	3,199
MADAGASCAR	155,000	0.0050	1,500	10	16	57	378
MALAWI	13,000	3.2680	115,000	–	641	177,630	27,215
MALAYSIA	–	0.1652	14,000	791	75	174	28,069
MALDIVES	720	–	–	–	446	–	36
MALI	–	0.0017	600	28	1,037	103	21
MALTA	–	–	–	285	347	–	25
MARSHALL ISLANDS	–	–	–	–	–	–	–
MAURITANIA	250	–	–	–	–	–	–
MAURITIUS	9,800	0.2540	298	392	1,236	35	87
MEXICO	–	0.0080	19,381	13,874	410	6,636	13,749
MICRONESIA, FEDERATED STATES OF	3,400	–	–	–	–	–	–
MOLDOVA, REPUBLIC OF	–	0.1867	4,850	197	5,320	4,875	2,057
MONACO	–	0.0027	–	–	–	–	–
MONGOLIA	200	–	–	4	1,207	–	–
MONTENEGRO	2,500	–	–	–	–	–	–
MOROCCO	7,900	–	4,300	0	2,722	0	4,242
MOZAMBIQUE	20,000	0.0175	11,000	0	127	39,242	4,728
MYANMAR	–	0.1668	35,000	–	–	–	–
NAMIBIA	–	–	–	498	1,060	2	111
NAURU	2,729	–	–	–	–	–	–
NEPAL	–	0.0711	2,718	0	–	–	–
NETHERLANDS	0	–	–	345,385	14,736	13,025	117,667
NEW ZEALAND	1,950	0.0000	0	744	2,555	128	1,636
NICARAGUA	970	0.0348	3,200	1	422	419	20
NIGER	23,000	0.0026	810	817	1,643	3	7
NIGERIA	–	0.0338	14,000	–	–	–	–
NIUE	–	–	–	–	–	–	–
NORWAY	900	–	–	30	2,201	–	2,182
OMAN	270	0.0150	–	1,934	2,172	79	0
PAKISTAN	62,000	0.1866	112,600	29	52	4,220	2,220
PALAU	–	–	–	–	–	–	–
PALESTINIAN TERR., OCCUPIED	1,500	0.2349	–	–	–	–	–
PANAMA	–	0.0583	2,600	2	729	252	7
PAPUA NEW GUINEA	8,200	–	–	12	0	–	–
PARAGUAY	690	0.0322	15,000	1,576	3,787	4,028	34,090
PERU	27,000	0.0031	2,300	0	3,830	1,770	–
PHILIPPINES	17,600	0.2425	38,368	16,965	401	19,043	65,021
POLAND	800	0.0935	38,411	40	3,120	15,178	76,785
PORTUGAL	–	0.0440	2,400	11,507	4,658	11,906	4,719
QATAR	1,400	–	–	16	2,001	0	4,861
ROMANIA	10	0.0222	1,686	9,149	3,347	1,136	20,759
RUSSIAN FEDERATION	2,800	0.0001	10	16,462	4,884	850	271,841
RWANDA	–	0.1443	3,800	0	323	–	252

3 Manufacturing	4 Price		5 Tax	6 WHO FCTC		7 Tobacco Industry Documents		COUNTRY
Cigarettes Manufactured (millions, 2007 or latest)	Marlboro or Equivalent (USD per pack)	Local Brand (USD per pack)	as a proportion of retail price	Signed	Ratified or acceded	on the Legacy Website 2008	Country Income Classification (World Bank, July 2008)	
–	–	–	40.28%	23-Jun-04	14-Jan-05	1,080	Lower middle	LESOTHO
25	$0.70	$0.70	14.00%	25-Jun-04	–	6,071	Low	LIBERIA
4,100	$1.79	$0.99	2.00%	18-Jun-04	7-Jun-05	3,662	Upper middle	LIBYAN ARAB JAMAHIRIYA
14,238	$1.71	$1.49	66.85%	22-Sep-03	16-Dec-04	5,969	Upper middle	LITHUANIA
–	$5.07	$4.86	70.10%	16-Jun-03	30-Jun-05	16,958	High	LUXEMBOURG
5,123	$0.69	$0.83	48.25%	–	30-Jun-06	23,956	Lower middle	MACEDONIA, FORMER YUGOSLAV REPUBLIC OF
4,979	$0.62	$0.75	63.67%	24-Sep-03	22-Sep-04	2,514	Low	MADAGASCAR
850	$0.57	$0.57	53.89%	–	–	25,425	Low	MALAWI
22,799	$2.34	$1.86	49.00%–5.007%	23-Sep-03	16-Sep-05	72,495	Upper middle	MALAYSIA
–	–	–	51.00%	17-May-04	20-May-04	1,006	Lower middle	MALDIVES
–	–	–	30.25%	23-Sep-03	19-Oct-05	53,603	Low	MALI
1,600	$3.55	$4.72	76.58%	16-Jun-03	24-Sep-03	10,719	High	MALTA
–	–	–	–	16-Jun-03	8-Dec-04	4,289	Lower middle	MARSHALL ISLANDS
–	–	–	20.28%	24-Jun-04	28-Oct-05	2,013	Low	MAURITANIA
650	$3.50	$3.50	82.04%	17-Jun-03	17-May-04	15,856	Upper middle	MAURITIUS
45,521	$1.98	$1.60	59.00%	12-Aug-03	28-May-04	115,186	Upper middle	MEXICO
–	–	–	–	28-Jun-04	18-Mar-05	840	Lower middle	MICRONESIA, FEDERATED STATES OF
5,031	$0.80	$0.16	24.40%	29-Jun-04	–	3,575	Lower middle	MOLDOVA, REPUBLIC OF
–	–	–	–	–	–	7,774	High	MONACO
–	–	–	40.09%	16-Jun-03	27-Jan-04	1,876	Lower middle	MONGOLIA
–	$1.73	–	56.00%	–	23-Oct-06	4,166	Upper middle	MONTENEGRO
11,158	$3.92	$1.80	66.67%	16-Apr-04	–	8,110	Lower middle	MOROCCO
1,800	$0.50	$0.50	50.53%	18-Jun-03	–	3,165	Low	MOZAMBIQUE
9,834	$0.31	$0.31	75.00%	23-Oct-03	21-Apr-04	12,536	Low	MYANMAR
–	–	–	42.40%	29-Jan-04	7-Nov-05	1,675	Lower middle	NAMIBIA
–	–	–	–	–	29-Jun-04	522	–	NAURU
7,736	$1.38	$0.97	81.50%	3-Dec-03	7-Nov-06	4,629	Low	NEPAL
85,440	$5.48	$4.59	74.49%	16-Jun-03	27-Jan-05	95,212	High	NETHERLANDS
756	$7.31	$7.08	69.11%	16-Jun-03	27-Jan-04	68,218	High	NEW ZEALAND
2,400	$0.61	$0.77	40.04%	7-Jun-04	9-Apr-08	18,222	Lower middle	NICARAGUA
–	$0.45	$0.45	32.25%	28-Jun-04	25-Aug-05	26,996	Low	NIGER
12,000	$1.55	$1.53	32.76%	28-Jun-04	20-Oct-05	35,286	Low	NIGERIA
–	–	–	–	18-Jun-04	3-Jun-05	2,230	–	NIUE
718	$11.48	$11.48	76.10%	16-Jun-03	16-Jun-03	50,849	High	NORWAY
–	$1.84	$1.59	40.50%	–	9-Mar-05	34,730	High	OMAN
62,073	$1.16	$0.86	69.00%	18-May-05	3-Nov-04	37,632	Low	PAKISTAN
–	–	–	–	16-Jun-03	12-Feb-04	810	Upper middle	PALAU
–	–	–	–	–	–	1,383	Lower middle	PALESTINIAN TERR., OCCUPIED
760	$1.30	$0.65	26.76%	26-Sep-03	16-Aug-04	41,572	Upper middle	PANAMA
50	$2.30	$1.85	–	22-Jun-04	25-May-06	5,669	Low	PAPUA NEW GUINEA
4,038	$0.99	$0.56	19.09%	16-Jun-03	26-Sep-06	11,976	Lower middle	PARAGUAY
1,422	$1.71	$1.64	34.97%	21-Apr-04	30-Nov-04	24,658	Lower middle	PERU
110,021	$0.61	$0.57	46.00%–49.00%	23-Sep-03	6-Jun-05	33,360	Lower middle	PHILIPPINES
130,272	$2.58	$2.34	87.06%	14-Jun-04	15-Sep-06	40,932	Upper middle	POLAND
21,972	$4.32	$4.18	79.60%	9-Jan-04	8-Nov-05	28,919	High	PORTUGAL
–	$1.35	$1.35	33.00%	17-Jun-03	23-Jul-04	6,650	High	QATAR
25,000	$1.91	$2.13	73.88%	25-Jun-04	27-Jan-06	14,810	Upper middle	ROMANIA
398,200	$1.62	$1.13	33.11%	–	3-Jun-08	64,339	Upper middle	RUSSIAN FEDERATION
–	–	–	65.25%	2-Jun-04	19-Oct-05	1,572	Low	RWANDA

TABLE B THE BUSINESS OF TOBACCO

COUNTRY	1 Growing Tobacco		2 Tobacco Trade				
	Tobacco Harvest Area (hectares, 2004–2007)	Agricultural Land under Tobacco (percent of total, 2005)	Tobacco Produced (metric tons, 2006)	Cigarette Exports (millions, 2002–2007)	Cigarette Imports (millions, 2004–2007)	Tobacco Leaf Exports (metric tons, 2006)	Tobacco Leaf Imports (metric tons, 2006)
SAINT KITTS AND NEVIS	–	–	–	–	–	–	–
SAINT LUCIA	70	–	–	–	–	–	–
SAINT VINCENT AND GRENADINES	50	–	85	–	–	–	–
SAMOA	–	–	140	0	0	–	–
SAN MARINO	–	–	–	–	–	–	–
SAO TOME AND PRINCIPE	–	–	–	–	–	–	–
SAUDI ARABIA	–	–	–	19	23,603	0	344
SENEGAL	8,043	–	–	1,783	1,190	855	2,687
SERBIA	–	0.1326	10,808	840	3,456	4,016	9,363
SEYCHELLES	60	–	–	–	–	–	–
SIERRA LEONE	0	0.0021	30	–	–	–	–
SINGAPORE	656	0.0000	–	20,518	16,326	2,024	19,017
SLOVAKIA	–	0.0481	668	19	6,152	1,553	1,558
SLOVENIA	100	–	–	0	5,698	–	71
SOLOMON ISLANDS	250	0.1176	85	–	–	–	–
SOMALIA	9,000	0.0006	–	–	–	–	–
SOUTH AFRICA	14,000	0.0090	17,500	9,497	1,307	13,368	28,807
SPAIN	2,680	0.0446	42,000	1,386	63,229	32,943	30,710
SRI LANKA	–	0.1290	3,710	116	101	–	–
SUDAN	–	–	–	–	–	–	4,502
SURINAME	200	–	–	–	–	–	–
SWAZILAND	–	0.0144	75	–	–	–	–
SWEDEN	550	–	–	195	7,158	35	4,081
SWITZERLAND	16,800	0.0447	1,270	47,137	615	3,848	30,751
SYRIAN ARAB REPUBLIC	1,600	0.1162	29,500	7	4,255	1,620	1
TAJIKISTAN	36,000	0.0277	–	–	–	–	–
TANZANIA, UNITED REPUBLIC OF	40,000	0.0990	52,000	58	56	37,525	849
THAILAND	–	0.2151	70,000	772	12,269	27,807	3,986
TIMOR-LESTE	17,200	–	–	–	78	–	–
TOGO	4,100	0.1102	1,800	32	1,627	–	–
TONGA	–	–	–	–	–	–	–
TRINIDAD AND TOBAGO	130	0.0977	200	3,776	15	–	505
TUNISIA	2,500	0.0229	3,500	2,553	2,879	321	7,085
TURKEY	146,000	0.4496	98,137	446	1	120,892	19,421
TURKMENISTAN	1,600	0.0048	3,500	–	–	–	–
TUVALU	–	–	–	–	–	–	–
UGANDA	18,000	–	32,000	243	1,389	16,023	186
UKRAINE	500	0.0015	340	–	–	2,006	74,408
UNITED ARAB EMIRATES	40	0.0054	–	39,075	20,852	469	197
UNITED KINGDOM	–	–	–	24,670	5,231	5,118	57,328
UNITED STATES OF AMERICA	144,068	0.0291	329,918	100,744	17,562	138,579	234,263
URUGUAY	900	0.0060	3,000	2,728	118	2,131	6,155
UZBEKISTAN	6,600	0.0233	20,000	–	–	–	–
VANUATU	–	–	–	–	–	–	–
VENEZUELA	3,600	0.0116	5,035	1,481	2	0	7,168
VIETNAM	27,000	0.1751	42,600	–	149	6,539	31,039
YEMEN	9,300	0.0458	20,200	4,659	155	32	8,937
ZAMBIA	4,500	0.1010	4,800	126	446	35,262	1
ZIMBABWE	51,800	0.3278	44,451	3,218	1,528	–	–

Cigarettes Manufactured (millions, 2007 or latest)	Marlboro or Equivalent (USD per pack)	Local Brand (USD per pack)	Tax as a proportion of retail price	Signed	Ratified or acceded	on the Legacy Website 2008	Country Income Classification (World Bank, July 2008)	COUNTRY
–	–	–	–	29-Jun-04	–	378	Upper middle	SAINT KITTS AND NEVIS
–	–	–	–	29-Jun-04	7-Nov-05	607	Upper middle	SAINT LUCIA
–	–	–	2.00%	14-Jun-04	–	184	Upper middle	SAINT VINCENT AND GRENADINES
–	–	–	–	25-Sep-03	3-Nov-05	2,530	Lower middle	SAMOA
–	–	–	–	26-Sep-03	7-Jul-04	1,130	High	SAN MARINO
–	–	–	22.66%–26.09%	18-Jun-04	12-Apr-06	239	Low	SAO TOME AND PRINCIPE
900	$1.51	–	38.18%	24-Jun-04	9-May-05	26,593	High	SAUDI ARABIA
5,000	$1.26	$0.84	36.25%	19-Jun-03	27-Jan-05	6,775	Low	SENEGAL
16,000	$1.73	$1.06	56.00%	28-Jun-04	8-Feb-06	4,014	Upper middle	SERBIA
–	–	–	60.71%–63.04%	11-Sep-03	12-Nov-03	1,475	Upper middle	SEYCHELLES
1,225	$0.85	$0.85	36.67%	–	–	13,080	Low	SIERRA LEONE
8,240	$7.63	$6.71	73.76%	29-Dec-03	14-May-04	72,337	High	SINGAPORE
50	$2.72	$3.01	93.55%	19-Dec-03	4-May-04	5,376	High	SLOVAKIA
438	$3.47	$1.93	74.85%	25-Sep-03	15-Mar-05	3,375	High	SLOVENIA
–	–	–	–	18-Jun-04	10-Aug-04	2,098	Low	SOLOMON ISLANDS
–	–	–	–	–	–	2,917	Low	SOMALIA
31,500	$2.69	$2.50	44.28%	16-Jun-03	19-Apr-05	80,932	Upper middle	SOUTH AFRICA
39,798	$4.04	$3.36	77.63%	16-Jun-03	11-Jan-05	85,307	High	SPAIN
4,150	$2.47	$2.12	67.04%	23-Sep-03	11-Nov-03	22,755	Lower middle	SRI LANKA
2,500	$2.40	$0.96	–	10-Jun-04	31-Oct-05	10,024	Lower middle	SUDAN
380	$1.82	$1.82	45.41%–47.09%	24-Jun-04	16-Dec-08	9,199	Upper middle	SURINAME
–	–	–	32.28%	29-Jun-04	13-Jan-06	1,991	Lower middle	SWAZILAND
5,700	$6.77	$6.63	72.25%	16-Jun-03	7-Jul-05	95,067	High	SWEDEN
53,164	$5.71	$5.29	62.60%	25-Jun-04	–	157,079	High	SWITZERLAND
15,300	$1.56	$0.68	25.00%	11-Jul-03	22-Nov-04	9,489	Lower middle	SYRIAN ARAB REPUBLIC
6,400	$0.50	$0.50	–	–	–	1,220	Low	TAJIKISTAN
4,550	$1.10	$0.81	36.67%	27-Jan-04	30-Apr-07	9,857	Low	TANZANIA, UNITED REPUBLIC OF
29,000	$1.75	$1.34	69.54%	20-Jun-03	8-Nov-04	41,000	Lower middle	THAILAND
–	–	–	–	25-May-04	22-Dec-04	1,141	Lower middle	TIMOR-LESTE
–	$1.08	$0.50	30.25%	12-May-04	15-Nov-05	5,027	Low	TOGO
–	–	–	–	25-Sep-03	8-Apr-05	1,356	Lower middle	TONGA
5,180	$2.28	$1.60	20.04%	27-Aug-03	19-Aug-04	43,368	High	TRINIDAD AND TOBAGO
13,800	$2.56	$0.86	67.00%	22-Aug-03	–	5,077	Lower middle	TUNISIA
101,000	$3.54	$3.08	58.00%	28-Apr-04	31-Dec-04	58,473	Upper middle	TURKEY
4,600	$1.30	$1.30	73.67%	–	–	1,355	Lower middle	TURKMENISTAN
–	–	–	–	10-Jun-04	26-Sep-05	337	–	TUVALU
2,300	$1.20	$1.20	71.25%	5-Mar-04	20-Jun-07	13,429	Low	UGANDA
128,531	$0.95	$0.79	34.89%	25-Jun-04	6-Jun-06	12,809	Lower middle	UKRAINE
–	$1.63	$1.48	31.90%	24-Jun-04	7-Nov-05	36,506	High	UNITED ARAB EMIRATES
7,800	$10.72	$8.24	76.49%	16-Jun-03	16-Dec-04	889,297	High	UNITED KINGDOM
484,000	$4.79	$4.75	36.93%	10-May-04	–	1,864,723	High	UNITED STATES OF AMERICA
5,458	$2.06	$1.93	87.36%	19-Jun-03	9-Sep-04	13,138	Upper middle	URUGUAY
8,000	$1.02	$0.44	62.00%	–	–	7,885	Low	UZBEKISTAN
–	–	–	–	22-Apr-04	16-Sep-05	489	Lower middle	VANUATU
16,600	$0.74	$0.70	50.28%	22-Sep-03	27-Jun-06	54,475	Upper middle	VENEZUELA
86,160	$0.97	$0.70	45.00%	3-Sep-03	17-Dec-04	25,165	Low	VIETNAM
11,392	$0.82	$0.82	47.00%	20-Jun-03	22-Feb-07	4,507	Low	YEMEN
400	$2.02	$1.46	60.89%	–	23-May-08	10,431	Low	ZAMBIA
2,500	$1.16	$1.25	47.04%	–	–	35,922	Low	ZIMBABWE

113

SOURCES

PART ONE: PREVALENCE AND HEALTH

Tobacco "death clock" shows almost 40 million dead (Update1). (2008, October 21). Bloomberg News.

CHAPTER 1:
TYPES OF TOBACCO USE

Boffetta P, Hecht S, Gray N, Gupta P, Straif K. (2008, July). Smokeless tobacco and cancer. *Lancet Oncology*, 9(7): 667–675.

Maziak W, Ward KD, Afifi Soweid RA, Eissenberg T. (2004, December). Tobacco smoking using a waterpipe: a re-emerging strain in a global epidemic. *Tobacco Control*, 13(4): 327–333.

National Cancer Institute. (N.d.). *Smokeless tobacco and cancer.* http://www.cancer.gov/cancertopics/smokeless-tobacco. Accessed August 19, 2008.

National Cancer Institute. *Smoking and cancer.* (N.d.). http://www.cancer.gov/cancertopics/tobacco. Accessed August 19, 2008.

National Cancer Institute, Centers for Disease Control and Stockholm Centre of Public Health. (2002). *Smokeless tobacco fact sheets.* http://cancercontrol.cancer.gov/tcrb/stfact_sheet_combined10-23-02.pdf. Accessed August 19, 2008.

Prignot J, Sasco A, Poulet E, Gupta P, Aditama T. (2008, July). Alternative forms of tobacco use. *International Journal of Tuberculosis and Lung Disease*, 12(7): 718–727.

World Health Organization. (1997). *Tobacco or health: A global status report.* Geneva: WHO.

World Health Organization. (1998). *Guidelines for controlling and monitoring the tobacco epidemic.* Geneva: WHO.

CHAPTER 2:
MALE SMOKING
Quote
Smoke gets in your eyes: In a country of smokers, a small group of artists tries to clear the air. (2000, August 30). *Prague Post.*

Text
Bekedam H. (2008). Foreword. In T.-W. Hu (ed.), *Tobacco control policy analysis in China: Economics and health* (pp. v–vii). Berkeley: University of California.

ERC. (2007). *World cigarette survey 2007.* London: ERC Group Plc.

Ezzati M, Lopez AD. (2003, September 13). Estimates of global mortality attributable to smoking in 2000. *Lancet*, 362(9387): 847–852.

Ibison D. (1992, October 16). Rothmans' joint deal opens heavenly gates. *Window, Hong Kong*: 4.

Jha P et al. (2008). A nationally representative case-control study of smoking and death in India. *New England Journal of Medicine*, 358: 1137–1147.

Scull R. Bright future predicted for Asia Pacific. (1986, September). *World Tobacco*: 35.

World Health Organization. (2008). *WHO report on the global tobacco epidemic, 2008: The MPOWER package.* Geneva: WHO. http://www.who.int/tobacco/mpower/mpower_report_full_2008.pdf. Accessed June 23, 2008.

Map and Symbols
WHO MPOWER Report. (2008). The 2008 MPOWER report served as the data source for estimates of age-standardized current cigarette smoking prevalence for all countries, except the following:

Australia — AIHW. (2007). *2007 National Drug Strategy Household Drug Survey.* http://www.aihw.gov.au/publications/index.cfm/title/10579. Accessed June 2009.

Bahamas — Pan American Health Organization. (1992). *Tobacco or health: Status in the Americas.* http://publications.paho.org/product.php?productid=280. Accessed August 27, 2008.

Bhutan — Ugen S. (2003, December 12). Bhutan: The world's most advanced tobacco control nation? *Tobacco Control*, 4: 431–433.

Burundi — Mahwenya P. (1998). Analyse de la situation actuelle du tabagisme au Burundi. (N.p.).

Djibouti — Hersi AH. (1999). *Tobacco-related problems in Djibouti.* (N.p.).

Germany — Jahrbuch Sucht. (2009) Deutsche Hauptstelle für Suchtfragen e.V., Geesthacht 2009, Chapter 2.2 by Thomas Lampert and Sabine Maria List (RKI).

Hong Kong — Hong Kong Department of Health. (2003). *General household survey, 2003.* Hong Kong Department of Health.

Macedonia, Former Yugoslav Republic of — WHO regional office for Europe, Tobacco control database. WHO Health for All Database. http://data.euro.who.int/tobacco// Accessed August 27, 2008.

Micronesia, Federated State of — Shmulewitz D. (2001). Epidemiology and factor analysis of obesity, type II diabetes, hypertension, and dyslipidemia (Syndrome X) on the Island of Kosrae, Federated States of Micronesia. *Human Heredity*, 51: 8–19.

Niue — Laugesen M. (2003). *Mission report on tobacco from Niue.* Harley Stanton. Personal communication.

Northern Ireland — Northern Ireland Statistics & Research Agency. (2008). *Continuous Household Survey.* http://www.csu.nisra.gov.uk/survey.asp140.htm. Accessed June 2009.

Palestinian Authority — Palestine Central Bureau of Statistics. (1997). *Country profiles on tobacco control in the eastern Mediterranean region.* http://www.emro.who.int/TFI/CountryProfile.htm. Accessed August 2008.

Papua New Guinea — Tobacco-free initiative Western Pacific Region. World Health Organization, Western Pacific Regional Office, 2000. *Country profiles on tobacco or health 2000.* http://www.wpro.who.int/NR/rdonlyres/751257EA-1037-4E62-98F7-EBEEE278ADAF/0/countryprofiles2000.pdf. Accessed September 16, 2008.

Qatar — Hamad Medical Centre survey. (1999). Reported in *Country profiles on tobacco control in the eastern Mediterranean region.*

San Marino — World Health Organization. (1997). *Tobacco or health: a global status report.* Geneva: WHO. http://whqlibdoc.who.int/publications/1997/924156184X_eng.pdf. Accessed August 2008.

Sudan — *Country profiles on tobacco control in the Eastern Mediterranean region.*

Turkmenistan — Piha T et al. (1993). Tobacco or health. *World Health Statistics Quarterly*, 46: 188–194.

Tuvalu — Tuomilehto J, Zimmet P, Taylor R, Bennet P, Wolf E, Kankaanpaa J. (1986). Smoking rates in the Pacific Islands. *Bulletin of the World Health Organization* 64(3): 447–456.

United Kingdom — Office for National Statistics. (2007). *Smoking and drinking among Adults, 2007.* http://www.statistics.gov.uk/downloads/theme_compendia/GHS07/GHSSmokingandDrinkingAmongAdults2007.pdf. Accessed June 2009.

United States — Cigarette smoking among adults, United States, 2006. (2007, November 9). *Morbidity and Mortality Weekly Report*, 56(44):1157–1161.

Yemen — Hadarani A. (1998). Sanaa University survey. *Country profiles on tobacco control in the Eastern Mediterranean region.*

Age-standardized smoking prevalence estimates for **Canada**, **Saint Vincent**, the **Grenadines**, **Singapore**, and **Timor-Leste** were extrapolated from available data.

Smoking Trends
Cigarette smoking among adults, United States, 2006. (2007, November 9). *Morbidity and Mortality Weekly Report*, 56(44): 1157–1161.

Early release of selected estimates based on data from the January–September 2007 National Health Interview Survey. (N.d.). http://www.cdc.gov/nchs/data/nhis/earlyrelease/200712_08.pdf. Accessed August 25, 2008.

Japan Ministry of Health statistics. (N.d.). http://www.health-net.or.jp/tobacco/product/pd100000.html.

Japan Ministry of Health statistics. (N.d.). http://www.health-net.or.jp/tobacco/product/pd090000.html.

National Statistics Online. (N.d.). Smoking habits in Great Britain. http://www.statistics.gov.uk/cci/nugget_print.sp?ID=313. Accessed July 17, 2008.

Top 20 Male
U.S. Census Bureau, International Data Base. Table 094. Midyear Population, by Age and Sex. URL: http://www.census.gov/ipc/www/idb/tables.html. Accessed December 7, 2008.

File Folder
Areas of opportunity for R. J. Reynolds — 18–24 year old smokers. (1980). http://legacy.library.ucsf.edu/action/document/page?tid=kfx62d00&page=4. Accessed July 2, 2008.

Wow: China
Central Intelligence Agency. (2008). *The world factbook: China.* https://www.cia.gov/library/publications/the-world-factbook/geos/ch.html#People. Accessed June 23, 2008.

WHO MPOWER Report. (2008).

CHAPTER 3:
FEMALE SMOKING
Quote
NYC health. (2007, March 19). NYC has 123,000 fewer female smokers now than in 2002. Press release. http://www.nyc.gov/html/doh/html/pr2007/pr017-07.shtml. Accessed July 8, 2008.

Text
Ezzati M, Lopez AD, Rodgers A, Murray CJL. (Eds.). (2004). *Smoking and oral tobacco use: Comparative quantification of health risks, global and regional burden of disease attributable to selected major risk factors.* WHO: Geneva. http://www.who.int/publications/cra/chapters/volume1/part4/en/index.html. Accessed June 23, 2008.

The female smoker market. http://tobaccodocuments.org/landman/03375503-5510.html. Accessed July 12, 2005.

RJ Reynolds. (1985). Younger adult female analysis. http://legacy.library.ucsf.edu/tid/tlx58d00/pdf. Accessed July 2, 2008.

Tobacco.org Quotes. http://www.tobacco.org/quotes.php?mode=listing&records_per_page=25&pattern=smaller+babies. Accessed July 7, 2008.

Virginia Slims 5-year plan. (1989). http://legacy.library.ucsf.edu/action/document/page?tid=aln75e00&page=2. Accessed July 2, 2008.

World Health Organization. (2007). *The European tobacco control report: 2007.* Copenhagen: World Health Organization. http://www.euro.who.int/document/e89842.pdf. Accessed July 8, 2008.

World Health Organization. (2008). *WHO report on the global tobacco epidemic, 2008: The MPOWER package.* Geneva: WHO. http://www.who.int/tobacco/mpower/mpower_report_full_2008.pdf. Accessed June 23, 2008.

Map and Symbols
WHO MPOWER Report. (2008). The 2008 MPOWER report served as the data source for estimates of age-standardized current cigarette smoking prevalence for all countries, except the following:

Australia — AIHW. (2007). *2007 National Drug Strategy Household Drug Survey.* http://www.aihw.gov.au/publications/index.cfm/title/10579. Accessed June 2009.

Bahamas — Pan American Health Organization. (1992). Tobacco or health: Status in the Americas. http://publications.paho.org/product.php?productid=280. Accessed August 27, 2008.

Bhutan — Ugen S. (2003, December 12). Bhutan: The world's most advanced tobacco control nation? *Tobacco Control*, 4: 431–433.

Burundi — Mahwenya P. (1998). Analyse de la situation actuelle du tabagisme au Burundi. (N.p.).

Djibouti — Hersi AH. (1999). Tobacco-related problems in Djibouti. (N.p.).

Germany — Jahrbuch Sucht. (2009) Deutsche Hauptstelle für Suchtfragen e.V., Geesthacht 2009, Chapter 2.2 by Thomas Lampert and Sabine Maria List (RKI).

Hong Kong — Hong Kong Department of Health. (2003). General household survey.

Macedonia, Former Yugoslav Republic of — WHO Regional Office for Europe. (N.d.). Tobacco control database. WHO Health for All Database. http://data.euro.who.int/tobacco/. Accessed August 27, 2008.

Niue — Laugesen M. (2003). *Mission report on tobacco from Niue*. Harley Stanton. Personal communication.

Northern Ireland — Northern Ireland Statistics & Research Agency. (2008). *Continuous Household Survey*. http://www.csu.nisra.gov.uk/survey.asp140.htm. Accessed June 2009.

Palestinian Authority — Palestine Central Bureau of Statistics. (1997). *Country profiles on tobacco control in the eastern Mediterranean region*. http://www.emro.who.int/ TFI/CountryProfile.htm. Accessed August 2008.

Papua New Guinea — Tobacco-free initiative Western Pacific region. (2000). Country profiles on tobacco or health, 2000. Manila: World Health Organization, Western Pacific Regional Office. http://www.wpro.who.int/NR/rdonlyres/751257EA-1037-4E62-98F7-EBEEE278ADAF/0/countryprofiles2000.pdf. Accessed September 16, 2008.

Qatar — Hamad Medical Centre survey. (1999). *Country profiles on tobacco control in the eastern Mediterranean region*.

San Marino — World Health Organization. (1997). Tobacco or health: A global status report. Geneva: World Health Organization. http://whqlibdoc.who.int/publications/1997/924156184X_eng.pdf. August 2008.

Solomon Islands — Tobacco-free initiative Western Pacific region. (2000). Country profiles on tobacco or health, 2000. Manila: World Health Organization, Western Pacific Regional Office. http://www.wpro.who.int/NR/rdonlyres/751257EA-1037-4E62-98F7-EBEEE-278ADAF/0/countryprofiles2000.pdf. Accessed September 16, 2008.

Sudan — *Country profiles on tobacco control in the eastern Mediterranean region*.

Turkmenistan — Piha T et al. (1993). Tobacco or health. *World Health Statistics Quarterly*, 46: 188–194.

Tuvalu — Tuomilehto J, Zimmet P, Taylor R, Bennet P, Wolf E, Kankaanpaa J. (1986). Smoking rates in the Pacific Islands. *Bulletin of the World Health Organization*, 64(3): 447–456.

United Kingdom — Office for National Statistics. (2007). *Smoking and drinking among Adults, 2007*. http://www.statistics.gov.uk/downloads/theme_compendia/GHS07/GHSSmokingandDrinkingAmongAdults2007.pdf. Accessed June 2009.

United States — Cigarette smoking among adults, United States, 2006. (2007, November 9). *Morbidity and Mortality Weekly Report*, 56(44):1157–1161.

Yemen — Hadarani A. (1998). Sanaa University survey. *Country profiles on tobacco control in the eastern Mediterranean region*.

Age-standardized smoking prevalence estimates for **Canada**, **Saint Vincent** and the **Grenadines**, **Singapore**, and **Timor-Leste** were extrapolated from available data.

Smoking Trends
Cigarette smoking among adults, United States, 2006. (2007, November 9). *Morbidity and Mortality Weekly Report*, 56(44): 1157–1161.

Early release of selected estimates based on data from the January–September 2007 National Health Interview Survey. (N.d.). http://www.cdc.gov/nchs/data/nhis/earlyrelease/200712_08.pdf. Accessed August 25, 2008.

Japan Ministry of Health statistics. http://www.health-net.or.jp/tobacco/product/pd100000.html

Japan Ministry of Health statistics. http://www.health-net.or.jp/tobacco/product/pd090000.html

National Statistics Online. (N.d.). Smoking habits in Great Britain. http://www.statistics.gov.uk/cci/nugget_print.asp?ID=313. Accessed July 17, 2008.

Top 20 Female
U.S. Census Bureau, International Data Base. Table 094. Midyear Population, by Age and Sex. URL: http://www.census.gov/ipc/www/idb/tables.html. Accessed December 7, 2008.

File Folder
Cullman J. *Face the Nation* (CBS), January 3, 1971.

Wow: Twelve Percent
Greaves L, Jategaonkar N, Sanchez S. (Eds.) (2006). Turning a new leaf: Women, tobacco, and the future. British Columbia Centre of Excellence for Women's Health (BCCEWH) and International Network of Women Against Tobacco (INWAT). Vancouver: British Columbia Centre of Excellence for Women's Health.

Wow: Female Smokers
Jha P et al. (2008). A nationally representative case-control study of smoking and death in India. *New England Journal of Medicine*, 358: 1137–1147.

CHAPTER 4: HEALTH PROFESSIONALS

Quote
World Health Organization. *The role of health professionals in tobacco control*. (2005). http://www.who.int/tobacco/resources/publications/wntd/2005/bookletfinal_20april.pdf. Accessed August 2005.

Text
Fiore MC et al. (2000). *Treating tobacco use and dependence. Clinical practice guideline*. US Department of Health and Human Services, Public Health Service.

Gorin SS. (2001). Predictors of tobacco control among nursing students. *Patient Education & Counseling*, 44(3): 251–262.

Martinez C et al. (2008). Barriers and challenges for tobacco control in a smoke-free hospital. *Cancer Nursing*, 31(2): 88–94.

Terasalmi E et al. (2001). Smoking habits of community pharmacists in 12 European countries and their attitudes towards non-smoking work. World Health Organization, EUR/01/5025372.

Warren CW, Jones NR, Chauvin J, Peruga A. (2008). Tobacco use and cessation counseling: Cross-country data from the Global Health Professions Student Survey (GHPSS), 2005–2007. *Tobacco Control*, published online May 12, 2008; doi:10.1136/tc.2007.023895.

World Health Organization. (2004). Code of practice on tobacco control for health professional organizations. http://www.who.int/tobacco/communications/events/codeofpractice/en/. Accessed August 2005.

Map
Borges A et al. (2008). Smoking habits of sixth year medical students and anti-smoking measures in Portugal. *Revista Portuguesa de Pneumologia*, 14(3): 379–390.

CDC. (2005). Tobacco use and cessation counseling: Global health professionals survey pilot study, 10 countries, 2005. *Mortality and Morbidity Weekly Report*, 54(20): 505–509.

Dumitrescu AL. (2007). Tobacco and alcohol use among Romanian dental and medical students: A cross-sectional questionnaire survey. *Oral Health and Preventive Dentistry*, 5(4): 279–284.

Rapp K et al. (2006). A cluster-randomized trial on smoking cessation in German student nurses. *Preventative Medicine*, 42: 443–448.

Rzenicki A et al. (2007). Frequency of smoking tobacco among the students of the last year of the Faculty of Health Sciences [abstract]. *Przeglad Lekarski*, 64(10): 786–790.

Siemiska A et al. (2006). Tobacco smoking among the first-year medical students [abstract]. *Pneumonologia i Alergologia Polska*, 74(4): 377–382.

Smith DR, Leggat PA. (2007a). An international review of tobacco smoking among dental students in 19 countries. *International Dental Journal*, 57: 452–458.

Smith DR, Leggat PA. (2007b). An international review of tobacco smoking among medical students. *Journal of Postgraduate Medicine*, 53(1): 55–62.

Smith DR, Leggat PA. (2007d). Tobacco smoking habits among a complete cross-section of Australian nursing students. *Nursing and Health Sciences*, 9: 82–89.

Tan YM, Goh KL, Muhidayah R, Ooi CL, Salem O. (2003). Prevalence of irritable bowel syndrome in young adult Malaysians: a survey among medical students. *Journal of Gastroenterology and Hepatology*, 18(12): 1412–1416.

Warren CW, Jones NR, Chauvin J, Peruga A. (2008). Tobacco use and cessation counseling: Cross-country data from the Global Health Professions Student Survey (GHPSS), 2005–2007. *Tobacco Control*; doi:10.1136/tc.2007.023895.

Symbols
Albania, **Argentina, Croatia, Egypt, Philippines, Uganda** — CDC. (2005).

Armenia, Bangladesh, Bolivia, Bosnia and Herzegovina, Brazil, Czech Republic, Ghana, India, Indonesia, Iraq, Republic of Korea, Lebanon, Lithuania, Myanmar, Peru, Russian Federation, Saudi Arabia, Serbia, Slovakia, Sri Lanka, Syrian Arab Republic, Thailand, Tunisia, Vietnam — Warren, Jones, Chauvin, and Peruga. (2008).

Australia— Smith and Leggat. (2007d).

Canada, Denmark, Iran, Israel, Italy, Japan — Smith (2007).

China, Colombia, Greece, Ireland, Pakistan, Spain, Turkey — Smith and Leggat. (2007b).

France, Hungary, Jordan, Netherlands, United Kingdom, United States of America — Smith and Leggat. (2007a).

Germany — Rapp. (2006).

Malaysia — Tan, Goh, Muhidayah, Ooi, and Salem. (2003).

Poland — Rzenicki et al. (2007).

Portugal — Borges et al. (2008).

Romania — Dumitrescu. (2007).

Percent of Countries
World Health Organization. (2008). *WHO report on the global tobacco epidemic, 2008: The MPOWER package*. Geneva: WHO.

Counseling Students
Warren, Jones, Chauvin, and Peruga. (2008).

File Folder
Lorillard Tobacco. (1963, July 2). Kent and the physician: Confidential report. Bates No. 84420545/0583A. http://legacy.library.ucsf.edu/tid/trp54c00. Accessed August 12, 2008.

Wows
Albania
Warren, Jones, Chauvin, and Peruga. (2008).

Spain
Martinez et al. (2008).

CHAPTER 5: BOYS' TOBACCO USE

Quote
McDonald P. (2004). *Oxford Dictionary of Medical Quotations*. Oxford: Oxford University Press.

SOURCES

Text
Centers for Disease Control and Prevention. (2008). *Global Youth Tobacco Survey (GYTS): Data results by country and year: India factsheet.* http://www.cdc.gov/tobacco/global/GYTS/factsheets/searo/2006/India_factsheet.htm. Accessed July 9, 2008

Currie C et al. (Eds). (2008). Inequalities in young people's health: HBSC international report from the 2005/2006 Survey. Health Policy for Children and Adolescents, No. 5. Copenhagen: World Health Organization Regional Office for Europe.

Heruti R, Shochat T, Tekes-Manova D, Ashkenazi I, Justo D. (2004). Prevalence of erectile dysfunction among young adults: Results of a large-scale survey. *Journal of Sexual Medicine*, 1(3): 284–291.

Millett C, Wen LM, Rissel C, Smith A, Richters J, Grulich A, de Visser R. (2006). Smoking and erectile dysfunction: Findings from a representative sample of Australian men. *Tobacco Control*, 15(2): 136–139.

Natali A, Mondaini N, Lombardi G, Del Popolo G, Rizzo M. (2005). Heavy smoking is an important risk factor for erectile dysfunction in young men. *International Journal of Impotence Research*, 17(3): 227–230.

Warren CW, Eriksen MP, Asma S. (2006). Patterns of global tobacco use in young people and implications for future chronic disease burden in adults. *Lancet*, 367: 749–763.

Warren CW, Jones NR, Peruga A, et al. (2008). Global youth tobacco surveillance, 2000–2007. CDC Morbidity and Mortality Weekly Report Summaries. (2008, January 25). *Surveillance Summaries* 57(1): 1–28. www.cdc.gov/mmwr/preview/mmwrhtml/ss5701a1.htm. Accessed June 30, 2008.

Warren CW, Riley L, Asma S, et al. (2000). Tobacco use by youth: A surveillance report from the Global Youth Tobacco survey project. *Bulletin of the World Health Organization*, 78: 868–876.

Map
Centers for Disease Control and Prevention. (2008). Global youth tobacco survey (GYTS): Data results by country and year. http://www.cdc.gov/tobacco/global/GYTS/results.htm. Accessed July 1, 2008

Hayman J, White V. (2006).
Smoking behaviours of Australian secondary students in 2005. Centre for Behavioural Research in Cancer, Cancer Control Research Institute, The Cancer Council Victoria, http://www.nationaldrugstrategy.gov.au/internet/drugstrategy/publishing.nsf/Content/E1B70590AD4EF56DCA257225000EDCE9/$File/mono59.pdf. Accessed May 26, 2009.

Hublet A, De Bacquer D, Valimaa R, Godeau E, Schmid H, Rahav G, Maes L. (2006). Smoking trends among adolescents from 1990 to 2002 in ten European countries and Canada. *BMC Public Health* 6: 280.

Warren, Jones, Peruga, et al. (2008).

World Health Organization. (2008). *European health for all database (HFA-DB). Country profiles.* http://data.euro.who.int/Default.aspx?TabID=2404. Accessed July 1, 2008.

The Power of Branding
Centers for Disease Control and Prevention. (N.d.). Global youth tobacco survey (GYTS) data sets. http://www.cdc.gov/tobacco/global/surveys.htm#gyts. Accessed August 6, 2008.

Countries with the Highest Smoking Rates
Warren, Jones, Peruga, et al. (2008).

Wows
Unless Smoking Trends Change
Warren, Riley, Asma, et al. (2000).

Eighty-six Percent of Youth
Global Youth Tobacco Survey Collaborative Group. (2002). Tobacco use among youth: A cross-country comparison. *Tobacco Control*, 11: 252–270.

About 50 Million
World Health Organization Western Pacific Regional Office. (2008). Regional statistics. http://www.wpro.who.int/information_sources/databases/regional_statistics/rstat_tobacco_use.htm. Accessed June 24, 2008.

CHAPTER 6: GIRLS' TOBACCO USE
Text
Akbartabartoori M, Lean ME, Hankey CR. (2005). Relationships between cigarette smoking, body size and body shape. *International Journal of Obesity*, 29(2): 236–243.

Arora M, Reddy KS, Stigler MH, Perry CL. (2008). Associations between tobacco marketing and use among urban youth in India. *American Journal of Health Behavior*, 32(3): 283–294.

Global Youth Tobacco Survey Collaborative Group. (2003). Differences in worldwide tobacco use by gender: Findings from the Global Youth Tobacco Survey. *Journal of School Health*, 73(6): 207–215.

Honjo K, Siegel M. (2003). Perceived importance of being thin and smoking initiation among young girls. *Tobacco Control*, 12: 289–295.

Iauco DN. (1985, July 23). RJ Reynolds internal memorandum: Younger adult female smoker: New brand opportunity. (Bates No. 504103122/3124). http://legacy.library.ucsf.edu/tid/rux58d00. Accessed July 8, 2008.

Warren CW, Jones NR, Peruga A, et al. (2008). Global youth tobacco surveillance, 2000–2007. CDC Morbidity and Mortality Weekly Report Summaries. (2008, January 25). *Surveillance Summaries* 57(1): 1–28. www.cdc.gov/mmwr/preview/mmwrhtml/ss5701a1.htm. Accessed June 30, 2008.

Map
Centers for Disease Control and Prevention. (2008). Global youth tobacco survey (GYTS): Data results by country and year. http://www.cdc.gov/tobacco/global/GYTS/results.htm. Accessed July 1, 2008.

Hayman J, White V. (2006). Smoking behaviours of Australian secondary students in 2005. Centre for Behavioural Research in Cancer, Cancer Control Research Institute, The Cancer Council Victoria, http://www.nationaldrugstrategy.gov.au/internet/drugstrategy/publishing.nsf/Content/E1B70590AD4EF56DCA257225000EDCE9/$File/mono59.pdf. Accessed May 26, 2009.

Hublet A, De Bacquer D, Valimaa R, Godeau E, Schmid H, Rahav G, Maes L. (2006). Smoking trends among adolescents from 1990 to 2002 in ten European countries and Canada. *BMC Public Health*, 6: 280.

Warren, Jones, Peruga, et al. (2008).

World Health Organization. (2008). European health for all database (HFA-DB: Country profiles. http://data.euro.who.int/Default.aspx?TabID=2404. Accessed July 1, 2008.

Common Reasons
International Network of Women Against Tobacco. (2005). European women and smoking: INWAT factsheets. http://www.inwat.org/inwatreports.htm. Accessed August 20, 2008.

The Power of Branding
Centers for Disease Control and Prevention. (N.d.). Global youth tobacco survey (GYTS) datasets. http://www.cdc.gov/tobacco/global/surveys.htm#gyts. Accessed August 6, 2008.

GYTS Surveyed Countries
Warren, Jones, Peruga, et al. (2008).

Wows
The Difference in Current Cigarette Smoking Rates
Warren CW, Eriksen MP, Asma S. (2006). Patterns of global tobacco use in young people and implications for future chronic disease burden in adults. *Lancet*, 367(9512): 749–753.

Ninety Percent of Youth
Global Youth Tobacco Survey Collaborative Group. (2002). Tobacco use among youth: A cross-country comparison. *Tobacco Control*, 11: 252–270.

CHAPTER 7: CIGARETTE CONSUMPTION
Quote
Tobacco firms won't be stubbed out. (2006, September 27). BBC Online. http://news.bbc.co.uk/2/hi/business/5384038.stm. Accessed June 23, 2008.

Text
ERC. (2007). *World Cigarettes 1: The 2007 Report.* Suffolk, England: ERC Statistics Intl Plc.

United Nations Department of Economic and Social Affairs Population Division. *World population prospects: The 2006 revision and world urbanization prospects: The 2005 revision.* http://esa.un.org/unpp. Accessed August 20, 2008.

Map
Central Intelligence Agency. (2007). *The world factbook 2007.* Washington, DC: Government Printing Office. https://www.cia.gov/library/publications/the-world-factbook/. Accessed June 19, 2008.

ERC. (2007).

Symbols
ERC. (2007).

Global Cigarette Consumption
1880–1960
McGinn AP. (July/August 1997). The nicotine cartel. *World Watch Magazine*, 10(4): 18–27.

Proctor RN. (2001). Personal communication.

1970–2020
Guindon EG, Boisclair D. (2003). Past, present and future trends in tobacco use. HNP discussion paper: Economics of tobacco control paper No. 6. Geneva: World Health Organization Tobacco Free Initiative.

World Cigarette Consumption
ERC. (2007).

File Folder
Why one smokes. (1969). First draft of annual report to Philip Morris board by VP for research and development. Bates No. 1003287836_7848. http://www.pmdocs.com/. Accessed June 23, 2008.

Wows
ERC. (2007).

Chapter 8: Health Risks
Quote
World Health Organization. (2008). *WHO report on the global tobacco epidemic, 2008: The MPOWER package.* Geneva: WHO. http://www.who.int/tobacco/mpower/mpower_report_full_2008.pdf. Accessed April 4, 2008.

Text
Global Smokefree Partnership. (2008). Global voices: Working for smokefree air, 2008 status report. Naples, Italy: Global Smokefree Partnership. http://www.globalsmokefree.com/gsp/ficheiro/report.pdf. Accessed May 1, 2008.

Rogers JM. (2008). Tobacco and pregnancy: Overview of exposures and effects. *Birth Defects Research (Part C)*, 8: 1–15. http://www3.interscience.wiley.com/journal/117948112/. Accessed April 15, 2008.

United States Department of Health and Human Services. (2004). The health consequences of smoking: A report of the surgeon general. Atlanta: U.S. Department of Health and Human Services, Centers for Disease Control and Prevention, Office on Smoking and Health. http://www.cdc.gov/tobacco/data_statistics/sgr/sgr_2004/00_pdfs/insidecover.pdf. Accessed April 11, 2008.

United States Department of Health and Human Services. (2006). The health consequences of involuntary exposure to tobacco smoke: A report of the surgeon general. Atlanta: U.S. Department of Health and Human Services, Centers for Disease Control and Prevention, Office on Smoking and Health. http://www.surgeongeneral.gov/library/secondhandsmoke/report/. Accessed April 16, 2008.

United States Department of Health and Human Services. (2008). Smoking and tobacco use: Health effects of cigarette smoking, fact sheet. Centers for Disease Control and Prevention, Office on Smoking and Health.

http://www.cdc.gov/tobacco/ data_statistics/fact_sheets/ health_effects/health_effects .htm. Accessed August 20, 2008.

Woloshin S, Schwartz LM, Welch HG. (2008). The risk of death by age, sex, and smoking status in the United States: Putting health risks in context. *Journal of the National Cancer Institute*, 100: 845–853. http:// jnci.oxfordjournals.org/cgi/ content/abstract/djn124. Accessed June 10, 2008.

File Folder
Roe FJC, Pike MC. Smoking and lung cancer. Confidential report. (1965). British American Tobacco Co. Bates Number 105453524. http://legacy .library.ucsf.edu/tid/snc34a99. Accessed October 22, 2008.

Wows
The Risk of Dying
Centers for Disease Control and Prevention. (2008). Smoking and tobacco use: Health effects of cigarette smoking, fact sheet. http://www.cdc.gov/tobacco/ data_statistics/Factsheets/ health-effects.htm. Accessed April 15, 2008.

Pregnant Women's Tobacco Use
Bloch M, Althabe F, Onyamboko M, Kaseba-Sata C, Castilla EE, Freire S, Garces AL, Parida S, Goudar SS, Kadir MM, Goco N, Thornberry J, Daniels M, Bartz J, Hartwell T, Moss N, Goldenberg R. (2008). Tobacco use and secondhand smoke exposure during pregnancy: An investigative survey of women in 9 developing nations. *American Journal of Public Health*, 98(4): published online ahead of print February 28, 2008.

Goudar SS, Kadir MM, Goco N, Thornberry J, Daniels M, Bartz J, Hartwell T, Moss N, Goldenberg R. (2008). Tobacco use and secondhand smoke exposure during pregnancy: An investigative survey of women in 9 developing nations. *American Journal of Public Health* 98(10): 1833–1840.

Smoking Increases the Risk
Bates MN, Khalakdina A, Pai M, Chang L, Lessa F, Smith KR. (2007). Risk of tuberculosis from exposure to smoke. *Archives of Internal Medicine*, 167(18): 335–342.

CHAPTER 9: SECONDHAND SMOKE
Quote
O'Neil J. (2006, June 28). A warning on hazards of secondhand smoke. *New York Times.* http://www.nytimes.com/ 2006/06/28/health/28smoke .html. Accessed April 25, 2008.

Text
Global Smokefree Partnership. (N.d.). The benefits of smokefree policies. http://www .globalsmokefreepartnership .org/evidence.php?id=27. Accessed October 4, 2008.

Global Youth Tobacco Survey Collaborative Group. (2006). A cross-country comparison of exposure to secondhand smoke among youth. *Tobacco Control*, 15: 4–19. http://tobaccocontrol .bmj.com/cgi/content/full/15/ suppl_2/ii4#BIBL. Accessed April 25, 2008.

National Cancer Institute. (2007). Cancer trends progress report — 2007 update. Bethesda, MD: National Cancer Institute, National Institute of Health, U.S. Department of Health and Human Services. http:// progressreport.cancer.gov/ doc_detail.asp?pid=1&did=200 7&chid=71&coid=712&mid=. Accessed April 25, 2008.

Map
Australian Institute of Health and Welfare. National Drug Strategy Household Survey 2004–detailed findings AIWH cat. no. PHE 66. Canberra: Australian Institute of Health and Welfare, 2005. http://www .aihw.gov.au/publications/index .cfm/title/10190. Accessed May 26, 2009.

BMA Board of Science. Breaking the cycle of children's exposure to tobacco smoke. London, BMA, 2007.

Centers for Disease Control and Prevention. Global Youth Tobacco Surveillance, 2000-2007. Morbidity and Mortality Weekly Report, January 25, 2008 / 57(SS01);1-21. http:// www.cdc.gov/mmwr/preview/ mmwrhtml/ss5701a1.htm. Access June 2, 2009.

Centers for Disease Control and Prevention. (N.d.). Global Youth Tobacco Survey Country Fact Sheets. http://www.cdc.gov/ tobacco/global/GYTS/ factsheets/afro/factsheets.htm. Accessed April 24, 2008.

Global Youth Tobacco Survey Collaborative Group. (2006).

Symbols
Centers for Disease Control and Prevention. (2005–2007). *Global Youth Tobacco Survey: Country Factsheets — African Region (AFRO).* http://www.cdc .gov/tobacco/global/GYTS/ factsheets/afro/factsheets.htm. Accessed April 24, 2008.

Global Youth Tobacco Survey Collaborative Group. (2006).

National Cancer Institute. (2007).

United States Department of Health and Human Services. (2006). The health consequences of involuntary exposure to tobacco smoke: A report of the surgeon general. Atlanta: U.S. Department of Health and Human Services, Centers for Disease Control and Prevention, Office on Smoking and Health. http://www .surgeongeneral.gov/library/ secondhandsmoke/report/. Accessed April 16, 2008.

Number of Deaths
Smoke Free Partnership. (2006). *Lifting the smokescreen: 10 reasons for a smoke-free Europe.* Belgium: European Respiratory Society, Cancer Research UK, Institute National du Cancer, European Heart Network. http://dev .ersnet.org/uploads/Document/ 46/WEB_CHEMIN_1554_ 1173100608.pdf. Accessed April 25, 2008.

Harm Caused
United States Department of Health and Human Services. (2006).

File Folder
Mathews J. (1996, April 18). Claps and a flap over RJR "learn to crawl" remark. *Washington Post*, D9.

Wows
Nonsmokers Exposed
United States Department of Health and Human Services. (2006).

There Is No Risk-Free Level
United States Department of Health and Human Services. (2006).

Smoking in the Home
Hill SC, Liang L. (2008). Smoking in the home and children's health. *Tobacco Control*, 17: 32–37. http://tobaccocontrol.bmj.com/ cgi/content/full/17/1/32. Accessed August 20, 2008.

After the Implementation
Fernando D et al. (2007). Legislation reduces exposure to second-hand tobacco smoke in New Zealand bars by about 90%. *Tobacco Control*, 16: 235–238. http://tobaccocontrol.bmj.com/ cgi/content/full/16/4/235. Accessed August 20, 2008.

CHAPTER 10: DEATHS
Quote
The Bible, King James Version. (1611). Revelation 6:8.

Text
Takala J. (2002). Introductory report: Decent work — safe work. XVIth World Congress on Safety and Health at Work.

International Labour Office, Geneva. http://www.ilo.org/ public/english/protection/ safework/wdcongrs/ilo_rep.pdf. Accessed August 13, 2008.

United States Department of Health and Human Services. (2006). The health consequences of involuntary exposure to tobacco smoke: A report of the surgeon general. Atlanta: U.S. Department of Health and Human Services, Centers for Disease Control and Prevention, Office on Smoking and Health. http://www.surgeongeneral .gov/library/secondhandsmoke/ report/. Accessed April 16, 2008.

World Health Organization. (2008). *WHO report on the global tobacco epidemic, 2008: The MPOWER package.* Geneva: WHO.

Map
Ezzati M, Lopez AD. (2003). Estimates of global mortality attributable to smoking in 2000. *Lancet*, 362(9387): 847–852. http://www.thelancet.com/ journals/lancet/article/ PIIS0140673603143383. Accessed May 24, 2008.

Projected Global Tobacco-Attributable Deaths
Mathers C, Loncar D. (2006). Projections of global mortality and burden of disease from 2002 to 2030. *PLoS Medicine*, 13(11): 2011–2024. www.plosmedicine .org. Accessed April 24, 2008.

Cumulative Tobacco-Related Deaths
Fitzpatrick C, World Health Organization, Tobacco Free Initiative. (2008, May 13). Personal communication.

Wows
In the United States
United States Department of Health and Human Services. (2006).

Tobacco Causes up to 90% of Lung Cancers
WHO MPOWER Report. (2008).

PART TWO: THE COSTS OF TOBACCO

Russian public health chief accuses tobacco firms of US-inspired "genocide." (2008, July 22). Interfax News Service. http://www.cdi.org/russia/ johnson/2008-136-5.cfm. Accessed December 8, 2008.

CHAPTER 11: COSTS TO THE ECONOMY
Quote
Tobacco-Free Kids. Justice Department Civil Lawsuit. http://www.tobaccofreekids .org/reports/doj. Accessed October 4, 2008.

Text
Miller VP, Ernst C, Collin F. (1999). Smoking-attributable medical care costs in the USA. *Social Science and Medicine*, 48(3): 375–391.

Tobacco Free Initiative (TFI). (2001). Overview: The global crisis. Prepared for the International Policy Conference on Children & Tobacco. http:// www.tobaccofreekids.org/ campaign/global/crisis.shtml. Accessed May 20, 2008.

World Health Organization. (2005). WHO Framework Convention on Tobacco Control. http://www.who.int/tobacco/ framework/WHO_FCTC_ english.pdf. Accessed January 2, 2008.

Map
Argentina, Chile — Cevallos D. (2008, June 4). Health–Latin America: Tobacco regulations as solid as smoke. http://www .ipsnews.net/news.asp?idnews =42657. Accessed June 9, 2008.

Australia — Monograph Series No. 64 - The Costs of Tobacco, Alcohol and Illicit Drug Abuse to Australian Society in 2004/05.

Bangladesh — World Health Organization. (2007, April). Tobacco-related illnesses: Impact of in Bangladesh. New Delhi: Regional Office for South East Asia.

Barbados — Lwegaba A. (2004, January). Excess health care cost associated with a low smoking prevalence, Barbados. *West Indian Medical Journal*, 53(1): 12–16. (Authors' calculation)

Bosnia and Herzegovina, Guinea, Kenya, Mongolia, Namibia, Nauru, Sao Tome and Principe, Serbia and Montenegro, Turkey, Yemen — Riper TV. The world's heaviest-smoking countries. (2007, December 4). http://www .forbes.com/business/2007/ 12/04/smoking-africa-asia-biz-cx_tvr_1203smoking.html. Accessed December 12, 2008.

Brazil — Iglesias R, Jha P, Pinto M, da Costa e Silva V, Godinho J. (2007, August). Tobacco control in Brazil. Washington, DC: World Bank.

Canada — Rehm J, Baliunas D, Brochu S, et al. (2006, March). The costs of substance abuse in Canada 2002: Canadian Centre on Substance Abuse.

China — Hu T-w, Mao Z, Shi J. (2007). Tobacco taxation and its potential economic impact in China: Bloomberg Global Initiative to Reduce Tobacco Use Project. (Unpublished)

SOURCES

Czech Republic — Ross H. (2004). Critique of the Philip Morris study of the cost of smoking in the Czech Republic. *Nicotine & Tobacco Research*, 6(1): 181–189.

Denmark — Rasmussen SR, Prescott E, Sorensen TIA, Soraard J. (2004). The total life-time costs of smoking. *European Journal of Public Health*, 14: 95–100. (Authors' calculation)

Egypt — Nassar H. (2003, March). The economics of tobacco in Egypt: A new analysis of demand. Washington, DC: International Bank for Reconstruction and Development/World Bank.

Estonia — Taal A, Kiivet R, Hu T-W. (2004, June). The economics of tobacco in Estonia. Washington, DC: International Bank for Reconstruction and Development/World Bank.

Finland — Pekurinen, M. (1999). The economic consequences of smoking in Finland, 1987–1995. Helsinki: Health Services Research.

France — Fenoglio P, Parel V, Kopp P. (2003, January). The social cost of alcohol, tobacco and illicit drugs in France, 1997. *European Addiction Research*, 9(1): 18–28.

Germany — Neubauer S, Welte R, Beiche A, Koenig H-H, Buesch K, Leidl R. (2006). Mortality, morbidity and costs attributable to smoking in Germany: Update and a 10-year comparison. *Tobacco Control*, 15: 464–471.

Hong Kong — McGhee SM, Ho LM, Lapsley HM, et al. (2006). Cost of tobacco-related diseases, including passive smoking, in Hong Kong. *Tobacco Control*, 15: 125–130.

Hungary — Szilágyi T (2004). Economic impact of smoking and tobacco control in Hungary. Budapest: GKI Economic Research Institute.

Iceland — Sigillum Universitatis Islandiae. (2000). Cost of smoking in Icelandic society 2000: Report to Tobacco Control Task Force. Haskola Islands: Sigillum Universitatis Islandiae.

India — Ministry of Health and Family Welfare, Government of India. (2004, November 25). Report on tobacco control in India. New Delhi, India: Ministry of Health and Family Welfare.

Indonesia — Barber S, Adioetomo SM, Ahsan A, Setyonaluri D. (2008). Tobacco economics in Indonesia. Paris:

International Union against Tuberculosis and Lung Disease.

Ireland — Madden D. (2003, September). The cost of employee smoking in Ireland. Dublin: University College.

Japan — Aguinaga Bialous S, Hoang M-A, Iso H, et al. (2004). Recommendations for tobacco control policy: Tobacco-Free Japan. Tokyo and Baltimore: Institute for Global Tobacco Control, Department of Epidemiology and Johns Hopkins Bloomberg School of Public Health.

Korea, Republic of — Kang HY, Kim HJ, Park TK, Jee SH, Nam CM, Park HW. (2003). Economic burden of smoking in Korea. *Tobacco Control*, 12: 37–44.

Mexico — Mexican Social Security Institute. (2007). The total annual cost of medical care attributed to tobacco use.

Myanmar — Kyaing NN. (2003). Tobacco economics in Myanmar. Washington DC: International Bank for Reconstruction and Development/World Bank.

Netherlands — Van Genugten MLL, Hoogenveen RT, Mulder I, Smit HA, Jansen J, de Hollander AEM. (2003). Future burden and costs of smoking-related disease in the Netherlands: A dynamic modeling approach. *Value Health*, 6: 494–499.

New Zealand — Cancer Society of New Zealand. (2004, September). What smoking costs. New Zealand: Cancer Society of New Zealand.

Nigeria — Daramola Z. (2007, November 12). FG hailed over move against tobacco coys. *Daily Trust*.

Norway — Sanner T. (1991). What does cigarette smoking cost society? *Tidskr Nor Laegerforen* 11: 3420–3422. [Data taken from Abstract]

Philippines — Quimbo SLA, Casorla AA, Miguel-Baquilod M, Medalla FM. (2007). The economics of tobacco and tobacco taxation (Philippines). UPecon Foundation and Department of Health.

Poland — Krzyanowska A, Gogowski C. (2004, February). Nikotynizm na wiecie: Nastepstwa ekonomiczne (The global nicotine addiction and its economic consequences). *Mened-Ser Zdrowia*, 98–103 (in Polish).

Russian Federation — Ross H, Shariff S, Gilmore A. (In press). *Economics of tobacco taxa-*

tion in Russia. Baltimore, MD: Bloomberg Initiative to Reduce Tobacco Use.

Singapore — Quah E, Tan KC, Saw SLC, Yong JS. (2002). The social cost of smoking in singapore. *Singapore Medical Journal*, 43(7): 340–344.

South Africa — The economics of tobacco control project, School of Economics, University of Cape Town. (1998, June 30). The economics of tobacco control in Southern Africa. Cape Town: Research for International Tobacco Control (RITC).

Spain — Ahn N, Molina JA. (2001, February). Smoking in Spain: Analysis of initiation and cessation. Fundación de Estudiosde Economía Aplicada. (FEDEA). http://www.fedea.es/pub/Papers/2001/dt2001-02.pdf. Accessed December 15, 2008.

Sweden — Bolin K, Lindgren B. (2007). Smoking, health-care cost, and loss of productivity in Sweden, 2001. *Scandinavian Journal of Public Health*, 35(2): 187–196.

Switzerland — *The Age Australia*. (2008, April 9). Switzerland remains smoking haven. http://news.theage.com.au/world/switzerland-remains-smoking-haven-20080409-24wg.html. Accessed December 13, 2008.

Thailand — Pongpanich S. (2006). A comparative analysis between present and future tobacco-related health care costs in Thailand: Submitted to Southeast Asia Tobacco Control Alliance (SEATCA). (Unpublished)

Ukraine — Ross H, Shariff S, Gilmore A. (In press). *Economics of tobacco taxation in Ukraine*. Baltimore, MD: Bloomberg Initiative to Reduce Tobacco Use.

United Kingdom — Parrott S, Godfrey C. (2004, April 17). Economics of smoking cessation. *BMJ*, 328(7445): 947–949.

United States of America — Centers for Disease Control and Prevention (CDC). Smoking attributable mortality, years of potential life lost, and productivity losses — United States, 2000 - 2004. MMWR. 2008;57(45):1226-8.

Uruguay — Carbajales AR, Curti D. (2006). Economía del control del tabaco en los países del Mercosur y Estados Asociados: Uruguay. Washington, D.C.: Pan American Health Organization. http://www.paho.org/Spanish/AD/SDE/RA/tab_estudios_Mercosur.htm. Accessed December 15, 2008.

Venezuela — Pan American Sanitary Bureau (1998). Cost-benefit analysis of smoking. Caracas: Pan American Health Organization.

Vietnam — Ross H, Trung DV, Phu VX. (2007, December). The costs of smoking in Vietnam: The case of inpatient care. *Tobacco Control*, 16(6): 405–409.

Total Economic Cost of Tobacco
Aguinaga Bialous S, Hoang M-A, Iso H, et al. (2004). Recommendations for tobacco control policy: Tobacco-free Japan. Tokyo, Baltimore: Institute for Global Tobacco Control, Department of Epidemiology, and Johns Hopkins Bloomberg School of Public Health. http://www.tobaccofree.jp/E/Full.html. Accessed October 4, 2008.

Centers for Disease Control and Prevention (CDC). (2005, July 1). Morbidity and Mortality Weekly Report. Annual smoking-attributable mortality, years of potential life lost, and productivity losses: United States, 1997–2001. http://www.cdc.gov/mmwr/preview/mmwrhtml/mm5425a1.htm. Accessed October 4, 2008.

Collins DJ, Lapsley HM. (2008). The costs of tobacco, alcohol and illicit drug abuse to Australian society in 2004/05. Canberra: Macquarie University, University of Queens, University of New South Wales. http://www.nationaldrugstrategy.gov.au/internet/drugstrategy/publishing.nsf/Content/mono64. Accessed October 4, 2008.

The economics of tobacco control project, School of Economics, University of Cape Town. (1998, June 30).

Fenoglio P, Parel V, Kopp P. (2003, January). The social cost of alcohol, tobacco, and illicit drugs in France, 1997. *European Addiction Research*, 9(1): 18–28.

Hu, Mao, and Shi. (2007).

KrzySanowska and Glogowski. (2004, February).

Nassar H. (2003, March). The economics of tobacco in Egypt: A new analysis of demand. Washington, DC: World Bank.

Average number of employee sick days per year for smokers and nonsmokers, Taiwan, 1999 Tsai SP, Wen CP, Hu SC, Cheng TY, Huang SJ. (2005). Workplace smoking related absenteeism and productivity costs in Taiwan. *Tobacco Control*, 14 (Supplemental I): i33–i37.

Cost of Fires
Hall JR. (2007). The smoking material fire problem. National Fire Protection Association: Fire Analysis and Research Division. http://www.nfpa.org/assets/files//PDF/OS.SmokingMaterials.pdf. Accessed September 2, 2008.

Leistikow BN, Martin DC, Milano CE. (2000). Fire injuries, disasters, and costs from cigarettes and cigarette lights: A global overview. *Preventive Medicine*, 31: 91.

File Folder
Arthur D. Little International/Philip Morris. (2001). Public finance balance of smoking in the Czech Republic. http://www.tobaccofreekids.org/reports/philipmorris/#czech. Accessed December 3, 2008.

Wows
China — Liu Y, Rao K, Hu T, Sun Q, Mao Z. (2006). Cigarette smoking and poverty in China. *Social Science and Medicine*, 63(11): 2784–2790.

CHAPTER 12: COSTS TO THE SMOKER
Quote
Thoreau HD. (1910). *Walden: Or, life in the woods*. Cambridge: Houghton Mifflin Co.

Text
Semba RD, de Pee S, Sun K, Best CM, Sari M, Bloem MW. (2008, October). Paternal smoking and increased risk of infant and under-5 child mortality in Indonesia. *American Journal of Public Health*, 98(10): 1824–1826. http://www.ajph.org/cgi/content/abstract/98/10/1824. Accessed October 4, 2008.

Map
Algeria, Argentina, Australia, Austria, Bahrain, Bangladesh, Belgium, Brazil, Brunei Darussalam, Bulgaria, Canada, Chile, China, Colombia, Costa Rica, Cote D'Ivoire, Czech Republic, Denmark, Ecuador, Egypt, Finland, France, Germany, Greece, Guatemala, Hong Kong, Hungary, Iceland, India, Indonesia, Iran, Islamic Republic of, Ireland, Israel, Italy, Japan, Jordan, Kazakhstan, Kenya, Korea, Democratic People's Republic of, Kuwait, Libyan Arab Jamahiriya, Luxembourg, Malaysia, Mexico, Montenegro, Morocco, Nepal, Netherlands, New Zealand, Nigeria, Norway, Oman, Pakistan, Paraguay, Peru, Philippines, Poland, Portugal, Qatar, Romania, Russian Federation, Saudi Arabia, Senegal, Serbia, Singapore, South Africa, Spain, Sri Lanka, Sweden, Switzer-

SOURCES

land, Syrian Arab Republic, Thailand, Turkey, Ukraine, United Arab Emirates, United Kingdom, United States of America, Uruguay, Uzbekistan, Venezuela, Vietnam, Zambia — Economist Intelligence Unit. (2007, December). Worldwide cost of living survey. http://eiu.enumerate.com/asp/wcol_WCOLHome.asp. Accessed March 3, 2008.

Albania, Armenia, Bolivia, Cameroon, Croatia, Cuba, Cyprus, Dominican Republic, El Salvador, Estonia, Ethiopia, Honduras, Iraq, Jamaica, Lao People's Democratic Republic, Latvia, Lebanon, Lithuania, Macedonia, Former Yugoslav Republic of, Madagascar, Moldova, Republic of, Nicaragua, Panama, Slovakia, Slovenia, Sudan, Tanzania, United Republic of, Togo, Trinidad and Tobago — ERC. (2007). *World cigarettes 1: The 2007 report*. Suffolk, England: ERC Statistics Intl Plc.

Afghanistan, Barbados, Belarus, Belize, Benin, Bosnia and Herzegovina, Burkina Faso, Burundi, Chad, Congo, Congo, Democratic Republic of the, Fiji, Guinea, Guyana, Haiti, Kyrgyzstan, Liberia, Malawi, Mauritius, Mozambique, Myanmar, Niger, Sierra Leone, Suriname, Tajikistan, Turkmenistan, Uganda, Yemen — TMA world cigarette guide, 2008. Revised September 1, 2008. Tobacco Merchants Association. http://www.tma.org/tmalive/Html/CompendiumsAll.htm. Accessed december 15, 2008.

Angola, Azerbaijan, Cambodia, Georgia, Ghana, Korea, Republic of, Malta, Papua, New Guinea, Tunisia, Zimbabwe — White A. (2004). *A pack of Marlboros costs...* Global Partnerships for Tobacco Control, Essential Action. http://lists.essential.org/pipermail/gptc/2004q2/000130.html Accessed December 15, 2008.

Symbols
Economist Intelligence Unit. (2008). Worldwide cost of living survey. http://eiu.enumerate.com/asp/wcol_WCOLHome.asp. Accessed March 3, 2008.

World Bank. (2008). *World development indicators 2008*. Washington DC: World Bank.

Hourly wage estimates were derived by dividing World Bank GNI per capita (Atlas method) by 2,080 hours (40-hour work-week, 52 weeks per year).

Average Price
Economist Intelligence Unit. (2008).

Price of 20 Marlboro Cigarettes
Economist Intelligence Unit. (2008).

Matlick D. (2008, January). An upbeat future. *Tobacco Reporter*.

Wows
Albania — Ross H, Zaloshnja E, Levy D, Tole D. (In review). Results from the Albanian Adult Tobacco Survey. *Central European Journal of Public Health*.

Bangladesh — World Health Organization. (2004). Tobacco and poverty: A vicious circle. http://www.who.int/tobacco/communications/events/wntd/2004/en/wntd2004_brochure_en.pdf. Accessed March 29, 2008.

Indonesia — Best CM, Sun K, de Pee S, Sari M, Bloem MW, Semba RD. (2008). Paternal smoking and increased risk of child malnutrition among families in rural Indonesia. *Tobacco Control*, 17: 38–45. doi:10.1136/tc.2007.020875.

PART THREE: THE TOBACCO TRADE

du Plessis J. (2008, August 1). Who's in the addiction business: Tobacco industry profits from old habits. *Electronic Telegraph* (UK).

CHAPTER 13: GROWING TOBACCO

Quote
Smoke gets in your eyes. (2004, July). *New Internationalist*. http://www.newint.org/features/2004/07/01/keynote/. Accessed August 14, 2008.

Text
Campaign for Tobacco Free Kids (2005). *Global leaf, barren harvest*. http://www.tobaccofreekids.org/campaign/global/FCTCreport1.pdf. Accessed August 19, 2008.

Christian Aid. (2002). Hooked on tobacco. Report by Christian Aid/DESER on British American Tobacco subsidiary, Souza Cruz. London: Christian Aid. http://212.2.6.41/indepth/0201bat/index.htm. Accessed June 11, 2008.

Christian Aid. (2004). Hooked on tobacco: BAT in Kenya. Behind the mask: The real face of corporate social responsibility. London: Christian Aid. http://212.2.6.41/indepth/0201bat/0401update.htm. Accessed June 11, 2008.

Food and Agricultural Organization. (N.d.a). FAOSTAT data, tobacco unmanufactured:

Production quantity, 2007; Area harvested, 2005; Agricultural area, 2005; Global tobacco production, 2005–2007. http://faostat.fao.org/site/567/DesktopDefault.aspx?PageID=567#ancor. Accessed August 14, 2008.

World Bank. (2008). Data and statistics: Country classification. http://web.worldbank.org/WBSITE/EXTERNAL/DATASTATISTICS/0,,contentMDK:20420458~menuPK:64133156~pagePK:64133150~piPK:64133175~theSitePK:239419,00.html. Accessed October 4, 2008.

Map
Food and Agricultural Organization. (N.d.b). FAOSTAT data, tobacco unmanufactured: Area harvested. http://faostat.fao.org/site/567/DesktopDefault.aspx?PageID=567#ancor. Accessed August 15, 2008.

Symbols
Food and Agricultural Organization. (N.d.b).

Food and Agricultural Organization. (N.d.c). *FAOSTAT data, agricultural area, 2005*. http://faostat.fao.org/site/377/DesktopDefault.aspx?PageID=377. Accessed April 16, 2008.

Global Tobacco Leaf Production
Food and Agricultural Organization. (N.d.b).

Leading Producers
Food and Agricultural Organization. (N.d.b).

Wows
China Produced
Food and Agricultural Organization. (N.d.b).

Four Countries
Food and Agricultural Organization. (N.d.b).

CHAPTER 14: TOBACCO COMPANIES

Quote
World's No. 2, 4 cigarette firms Rothmans, BAT announce merger. (1999, January 12). *Turkish Daily News*, Economy section. http://arama.hurriyet.com.tr/arsivnews.aspx?id=-511184. Accessed November 25, 2008.

Text
CNTC: Euromonitor International. (2007). The world market for tobacco. Dublin: Euromonitor International.

ERC. (2007). *World cigarettes 1: The 2007 report*. ERC Statistics Intl. Plc.

World Bank. (2008). *World development indicators 2008*. Washington DC: World Bank.

Map
ERC. (2007).

Symbols
Altria Group. (2008). About Altria. http://www.altria.com/about_altria/1_1_altriagroup.asp. Accessed October 15, 2008.

British American Tobacco. (N.d.). http://www.bat.com/group/sites/uk__3mnfen.nsf/vwPagesWebLive/DO52AD6H?opendocument&SKN=1. Accessed November 25, 2008.

Imperial Tobacco. (2008). Contact us. http://www.imperial-tobacco.com/index.asp?page=46. Accessed October 15, 2008.

Japan Tobacco Inc. (2008). Company profile. http://www.jti.co.jp/JTI_E/outline/gaiyou.html. Accessed October 15, 2008.

Phillip Morris International. (2008). Where to find us. http://www.philipmorrisinternational.com/PMINTL/pages/eng/ourbus/Where_to_find_us.asp. Accessed October 15, 2008.

Global Cigarette Market Share
CNTC: Euromonitor International. (2007).

All others: Connect-World. (N.d.). http://www.connect-world.net/Global_Themes/Health/Tobacco.html. Accessed August 20, 2008.

Tobacco Company Profits
Altadis Group. (2006). Annual report: Consolidated balance sheets. http://www.imperial-tobacco.com/files/altadis/reports/2006AR-En.pdf. Accessed November 25, 2008.

Altria/Philip Morris. (2006). Annual report: Financial review, consolidated statement of earnings. http://www.altria.com/AnnualReport/ar2006/2006ar_07_0500_01.aspx. Accessed October 15, 2008.

British American Tobacco. (2006). Annual review: Group income statement. http://www.bat.com/group/sites/uk__3mnfen.nsf/vwPagesWebLive/DO52AK34/$FILE/medMD6ZPK25.pdf?openelement. Accessed November 25, 2008.

Imperial Tobacco. (2006). Annual report: Financial highlights. http://www.imperial-tobacco.com/files/financial/reports/ar2006/files/IMT_2006_Report.pdf. Accessed October 15, 2008.

Japan Tobacco. (2006). Annual report: Consolidated statements of operations, Japan Tobacco Inc. and consolidated subsidiaries. http://www.jti.co.jp/JTI_E/IR/06/annual2006/

annual2006_E_all.pdf. Accessed October 15, 2008.

File Folder
Brown & Williamson, RJR merger approved. (2004, July 29). All-Business.com. http://www.allbusiness.com/retail-trade/food-stores/4482805-1.html. Accessed September 3, 2008.

CHAPTER 15: TOBACCO TRADE

Text
Boriss H, Kreith M. (2007). Commodity profile: Tobacco. University of California, Davis: Agricultural Issues Center. http://www.agmrc.org/NR/rdonlyres/7414D6C1-5DF1-46E2-AA78-B057E3259358/0/Tobacco2007.pdf. Accessed May 2008.

Hu, T. (2006, September 20). Balancing interests: The economics of tobacco control in China. *China Brief*, 6(19). http://www.jamestown.org. Accessed May 2008.

Otañez MG, Mamudu H, Glantz SA. (2007). Global leaf companies control the tobacco market in Malawi. *Tobacco Control*, 16: 261–269. http://tobaccocontrol.bmj.com/cgi/content/abstract/16/4/261. Accessed June 27, 2008.

Philip Morris. (1996). Trade. PM2047623773/3778. http://www.pmdocs.com/PDF/2047623773_377. Accessed May 22, 2008.

United Nations Statistics Division. (2008). United Nations Commodity Trade Statistics Database (COMTRADE). http://comtrade.un.org/db/dqBasicQueryResults.aspx?cc=240220&px=H2&r=ALL&y=2004,2005,2006,2007&p=0&rg=1&so=9999&qt=n. Accessed July 27, 2008.

United States Department of Agriculture, Economic Research Service. (2007). Tobacco outlook. http://usda.mannlib.cornell.edu/usda/ers/TBS//2000s/2007/TBS-04-24-2007.pdf. Accessed May 9, 2008.

World Health Organization. (2004). The millennium development goals and tobacco control. http://www.who.int/tobacco/publications/mdg_final_for_web.pdf. Accessed May 2008.

World Health Organization. (2008). *WHO report on the global tobacco epidemic, 2008: The MPOWER package*. Geneva: WHO. http://www.who.int/tobacco/mpower/mpower_report_full_2008.pdf. Accessed April 4, 2008.

SOURCES

Yach D, Wipfli H. (2006). A century of smoke. *Annals of Tropical Medicine & Parasitology*, 100(5): 465–479.

Map
United Nations Statistics Division. (2008a). Commodity Trade Statistics Database (COMTRADE). http://comtrade.un.org/db/dqBasicQuery Results.aspx?cc=240220&px=H2&r=ALL&y=2004,2005,2006,2007&p=0&rg=1&so=9999&qt=n. Accessed July 27, 2008.

Symbols
Top 5 Importing Countries
United Nations Statistics Division. (2008b). Commodity Trade Statistics Database, (COMTRADE). http://comtrade.un.org/db/dqBasicQuery Results.aspx. Accessed July 21, 2008.

Top 5 Exporting Countries
United Nations Statistics Division. (2008b).

Top 10 Exporters
United Nations Statistics Division. (2008c). Commodity Trade Statistics Database, (COMTRADE). http://comtrade.un.org/db/ce/ceSearch.aspx. Accessed May 27, 2008.

Top 10 Importers
United Nations Statistics Division. (2008c).

Cigarette Export Trade
Guindon GE, Boisclair D. (2005, August). Cigarette consumption dataset 1970–2004. Prepared for the American Cancer Society.

United Nations Statistics Division. (2008e). Commodity Trade Statistics Database, (COMTRADE). http://comtrade.un.org/db/dqQuickQuery.aspx. Accessed July 29, 2008.

Tobacco Leaf Export Volume
Guindon GE, Boisclair D. (2005, August). Cigarette consumption dataset 1970–2004. Prepared for the American Cancer Society.

United Nations Statistics Division. (2008e).

File folder
Gilmore AB, McKee M. (2004). Moving east: How the transnational tobacco industry gained entry to the emerging markets of the former Soviet Union. Part 1: Establishing cigarette imports. *Tobacco Control*, 13: 143–150.

Wow
United States Department of Agriculture, Economic Research Service. (2007). *Tobacco Outlook*. http://usda.mannlib.cornell.edu/usda/current/TBS/TBS-

10-24-2007.pdf. Accessed May 9, 2008.

CHAPTER 16: ILLEGAL CIGARETTES
Text
Action on Smoking and Health, UK. (2007). Essential information on tobacco smuggling .http://www.ash.org.uk/files/documents/ASH_122.pdf. Accessed October 2, 2008.

Colling J, LeGresley E, MacKenzie R, Lawrence S, Lee K. (2004). Complicity in contraband: British American Tobacco and cigarette smuggling in Asia. *Tobacco Control*, 13(Supplement II): ii104–ii111.

Framework Convention Alliance for Tobacco Control. (2007). COP-2 recommendations: A protocol on illicit trade in tobacco products. http://fctc.org/dmdocuments/fca-2007-cop-illicit-trade-cop2-recommendations-en.pdf. Accessed September 2, 2008.

Framework Convention Alliance for Tobacco Control. (2008). Glossary of terms in the illicit trade in tobacco products. http://www.fctc.org/dmdocuments/glossary_fact_sheet2.pdf. Accessed November 25, 2008.

Kohl, Hatch introduce bill to halt contraband cigarette trafficking linked to terrorist funding. (2003, June 6). http://www.tobacco.org/quotes.php?mode=listing&pattern=&records_per_page=200&starting_at=1800. Accessed March 3, 2008.

Tobacco News and Information. (N.d.). http://www.tobacco.org/quotes.php?starting_at=75. Accessed March 3, 2008.

Map
Barber S, Adioetomo SM, Ahsan A, Setyonaluri, D. (2008). *Tobacco economics in Indonesia*. Paris: International Union against Tuberculosis and Lung Disease.

Brazilian Ministry of Finance. (2007). Facts and figures on illicit trade in tobacco products. Unpublished data.

Ciecierski C, Weresa M, Jarczewska-Romaniuk A, Nakonieczna J, Filus L, Stoklosa M. (2008). *The economics of tobacco and tobacco taxation in Poland*. Paris: International Union Against Tuberculosis and Lung Disease.

ERC. (2006). *World cigarettes: The 2006 report*. ERC Statistics Intl. Plc.

ERC. (2007). *World cigarettes 1: The 2007 report*. ERC Statistics Intl. Plc.

Euromonitor International. (2005). *The world market for tobacco*. Euromonitor International Inc.

Euromonitor International. (2006). *The world market for tobacco*. Euromonitor International Inc.

Euromonitor International. (2007). *The world market for tobacco*. Euromonitor International Inc.

Framework Convention Alliance (2007). How big was the global illicit tobacco trade problem in 2006? Presented at the Conference of the Parties to the WHO Framework Convention on Tobacco Control, Bangkok, Thailand. http://www.fctc.org/dmdocuments/fca-2007-cop-illicit-trade-how-big-in-2006-en.pdf. Accessed November 25, 2008.

Gary G. (2008, January). Sine qua non. *Tobacco Reporter Magazine*. http://www.tobaccoreporter.com/home.php?id=119&cid=4&article_id=10719. Accessed September 2, 2008.

Kelly J. (2008, April). *Tackling tobacco smuggling in the UK*. PowerPoint presentation. Personal communication.

Lakhdar BC. (2008). Quantitative and qualitative estimates of cross-border tobacco shopping and tobacco smuggling in France. *Tobacco Control*, 17: 12–16.

Merriman D, Yurekli A, Chaloupka, F. (2000). How big is the worldwide cigarette smuggling problem? Pages 365–392 in *Tobacco control in developing countries*. P. Jha and F. Chaloupka. (Eds.). Oxford: Oxford University Press.

Paruyr A. (2006). Tobacco smuggling in Armenia. Unpublished manuscript.

Ross H, Shariff S, Gilmore A. (In press). *Economics of tobacco taxation in Russia*. Baltimore: Bloomberg Initiative to Reduce Tobacco Use.

Subuctageen A. (2006, September). Illegal tobacco trade in Pakistan. Presented at the first meeting of the WHO expert committee on the illicit tobacco trade, Geneva.

Verband der Cigarettenindustrie (2005), Bericht zur VdC-Studie Sammlung weggeworfener Cigarettenpackungen (EDP-Studie), VdC, Berlin.

World Health Organization. (2007). The European tobacco control report 2007. WHO Regional Office for Europe. http://www.euro.who.int/

Document/E89842.pdf. Retrieved July 30, 2008.

Seizures of Illicit Shipments
World Customs Organization. (2006). Customs and tobacco report 2006. Brussels.

Seizures of Cigarettes
HM Revenue and Customs. (2007. December). Annual performance report 2007 presented to Parliament by the financial secretary to the treasury by command of Her Majesty.

Evading Duty
Framework Convention Alliance (2007).

Recommendations
World Health Organization. (2007). Intergovernmental Negotiating Body on a Protocol on Illicit Trade in Tobacco Products, Conference of the Parties to the WHO Framework Convention on Tobacco Control. http://www.who.int/gb/fctc/PDF/it1/FCTC_COP_INB_IT1_4-en.pdf. Accessed September 16, 2008.

Wow
Schneider J. (2008, July). Imperial, Rothmans agree to pay C$1.15 billion over smuggling. http://www.bloomberg.com/apps/news?pid=20601082&sid=aypl.NwNN6rM&refer=canada. Accessed September 17, 2008.

PART FOUR: PROMOTION
Exhibit on cigarette advertising opens in NYC, "makes you want to smoke." (2008, October 9). Canadian Press. Quoting Dr. Robert Jackler, an associate dean of continuing medical education at Stanford University and curator of the tobacco ad exhibit at the NY Public Library.

CHAPTER 17: MARKETING
Quote
American Legacy Foundation. (2008). New research indicates cigarette makers manipulate menthol levels to attract young smokers. http://www.americanlegacy.org/2592.aspx. Accessed August 30, 2008.

Text
Big tobacco, lawless as ever. (2006, September 5). *Washington Post*. http://www.washingtonpost.com/wp-dyn/content/article/2006/09/04/AR2006090400947.html. Accessed September 30, 2008.

Charlesworth A, Glantz SA. (2005). Smoking in the movies increases adolescent smoking: A review. *Pediatrics*, 116(6): 1516–1528.

Polansky JR, Glantz S. (2007). *First-run smoking presentations

in U.S. movies, 1999–2006*. San Francisco: Center for Tobacco Control Research and Education.

Smoke Free Movies. http://www.smokefreemovies.ucsf.edu/index.html. Accessed July 10, 2008.

Tobacco: Global industry guide. (2008). London: Datamonitor.

U.S. Federal Trade Commission cigarette report for 2004 and 2005. (2007). Washington, DC: U.S. Federal Trade Commission.

Map
ERC. (2007). World cigarettes 1: The 2007 report. ERC Statistics Intl. Plc.

Marketing Expenditures
Frank Chaloupka. (2008, June 17). Personal communication.

Top-Selling Cigarette Brands
Japan Tobacco Inc. (2007). Annual report. http://www.jti.co.jp/JTI_E/IR/07/annual2007/annual2007_E_all.pdf. Accessed June 16, 2008.

Marketing Expenditures by Category
Chaloupka. (2008).

Silver Screen
Polansky & Glantz. (2007).

Wows
Of Hollywood's Top-Grossing
Brand identification: Wink, wink, nudge, nudge. (2008). http://www.smokefreemovies.ucsf.edu/problem/brand_id.html. Accessed July 14, 2008.

Big Tobacco's Marketing Experts
Big tobacco companies know the power of movies. (2008). http://www.smokefreemovies.ucsf.edu/problem/moviessell.html. Accessed July 10, 2008.

Today's 18-Year-Olds
Written direct examination of Michael Eriksen, ScD. (2005). *United States of America vs. Philip Morris USA, Inc.* Civil Action No. 99-CV-02496 (GK). www.usdoj.gov/civil/cases/tobacco2/01_Eriksen%20FINAL%20Written%20Direct%20Testimony.pdf. Accessed August 30, 2008.

CHAPTER 18: BUYING INFLUENCE
Quotes
Dr. Brawley
Harris G. (2008, March 26). Cigarette company paid for lung cancer study. *New York Times*. http://www.nytimes.com/2008/03/26/health/research/26lung.html. Accessed September 2, 2008.

Dr. Koop
Pekkanen J. (2007, December 1). Thank you for smoking.

Washingtonian. http://www .washingtonian.com/articles/ people/5856.html. Accessed September 2, 2008.

Text
Bero LA, Glantz S, Hong M-K. (2005). The limits of competing interest disclosures. *Tobacco Control*, *14*: 118–126.

Sylvester K. (1989, May). The tobacco industry will walk a mile to stop an anti-smoking law. *Governing*. http://www .governing.com/archive/1989/ may/tobacco.txt. Accessed September 25, 2008.

Tobacco-Free Kids and Common Cause. (2007). Campaign contributions by tobacco interests: Annual report: September 2007. http://tobaccofreeaction .org/contributions/Report _2007_09/Contributions_ 2007_09.pdf. Accessed May 19, 2008. Tobacco-Free Kids and Common Cause. (2007).

Buying Favors
Tobacco-Free Kids and Common Cause. (2007).

Buying Influence
Tobacco-Free Kids and Common Cause. (2007).

File Folders
Asia — Philip Morris Asia Corporate Affairs Plan, 1990–1992. (1989, December). Bates Number 2500084000/4042. http://legacy.library.ucsf.edu/ tid/lil19e00. Accessed September 2, 2008.

Kenya — Agriconsult. (1991, March). The economic impact of the tobacco industry in Kenya. Cited in Kweyuh P. (1994). Tobacco expansion in Kenya — the socio-ecological losses. *Tobacco Control*, *3*: 248–251. http://tobaccocontrol.bmj.com. Accessed September 25, 2008.

Philippines — Dollisson J. (1989, June 15). Second revised forecast presentation, Philip Morris corporate affairs. Bates Number 2500101311/1323. http://legacy.library.ucsf.edu/ tid/fml19e00. Accessed September 2, 2008.

United Kingdom — Langley A. (2003, May 20). Anti-tobacco pact gains despite firms' lobbying. *New York Times*. www .tobacco.org/quotes.php?mode= listing&pattern=betteridge& records_per_page=25. Accessed May 23, 2008.

United States — Report: Tobacco industry woos Connecticut lawmakers. (2003, August 23). Associated Press. www.tobacco.org/quotes .php?mode=listing&pattern=si

ngleton&records_per_page=25. Accessed May 23, 2008.

The Tobacco Institute
Sylvester. (1989).

CHAPTER 19: TOBACCO INDUSTRY
Quote
Victory for BAT in Australian cancer case. (2002, December 6). *Financial Times* (UK). http:// www.tobacco.org/quotes .php?mode=listing&pattern= harper&records_per_page=25. Accessed May 30, 2008.

Text
Legacy Library. (N.d.). http:// legacy.library.ucsf.edu. Accessed June 3, 2008.

Legacy Foundation. (N.d.). http://www.americanlegacy .org/awards/about.html. Accessed May 30, 2008.

Tobacco Archives. (N.d.). http:// www.tobaccoarchives.com/ maininfosettle.html. Accessed August 18, 2008.

Map
Legacy Library. (2008). http:// legacy.library.ucsf.edu/. Accessed August 3, 2008.

Top 5 Countries
Legacy. (2008). Number of tobacco industry documents by country. http://legacy.library .ucsf.edu/. Accessed June 3, 2008.

File Folders
Altria
New push grows for FDA regulation of tobacco. (2007, February 17). *Washington Post*. http://www.tobacco.org/quotes .php?mode=listing&pattern= parrish&records_per_page=25. Accessed May 30, 2008.

BAT Malawi
Illegal imports affect cigarette sales in Malawi. (2000, September 3). All-Africa.com/Pan African News Agency, http:// www.tobacco.org/quotes.php? mode=listing&pattern=faga& records_per_page=25. Accessed June 3, 2008.

BAT Nigeria
Tobacco giants "targeted African children to boost flagging profits." (2007, July 4). *Times of London* (UK). http://www .tobacco.org/quotes.php?mode= listing&pattern=Nigeria& records_per_page=25. Accessed May 29, 2008.

Philip Morris U.S.
U.S. trial against tobacco industry opens. (2004, September 22). *Washington Post*. http://www .tobacco.org/quotes.php?mode= listing&pattern=Ohlemeyer& records_per_page=25. Accessed May 29, 2008.

R.J. Reynolds
Russian financial woes take a toll in cigarettes. (1998, December 31). *New York Times*. http://www.tobacco.org/quotes .php?mode=listing&pattern= russia&records_per_page=25. Accessed June 3, 2008.

Philip Morris International
Philip Morris International. (29 March 1985). *The perspective of PM International on smoking and health issue*. Internal presentation. Bates Number 2023268329/8337. http:// legacy.library.ucsf.edu/tid/ nky74e00. Accessed December 15, 2008.

Wow
Taketa R. (2008, May 21). Personal communication.

PART FIVE: TAKING ACTION

WHO wants total ban on tobacco advertising. (2008, May 30). World Health Organization, quoting Dr. Douglas Bettcher, director of WHO's Tobacco Free Initiative, which has issued a call for a worldwide ban on all tobacco advertising, promotion, and sponsorship.

CHAPTER 20: RESEARCH
Quote
Warner KE. (2007, December). Charting the science of the future where tobacco-control research must go. *American Journal of Preventive Medicine*, *33*(6 Suppl): S314–S317.

Text
Baris E et al. (2000). Research priorities for tobacco control in developing countries: A regional approach to a global consultative process. *Tobacco Control*, *9*: 217–223.

Bero LA, Glantz S, Hong M-K. (2005). The limits of competing interest disclosures. *Tobacco Control*, *14*: 118–126.

Cohen JE. (2001). Universities and tobacco money. *BMJ*, *323*(7303): 1–2.

Grimm D. (2005). Is tobacco research turning over a new leaf? *Science*, *307*(5706): 36–37.

Rose JE. (2005). Ethics of tobacco company funding [letter]. *Science*, *308*(5772): 632.

Map
Europe — Schaap MM et al. (2008). Effect of nation-wide tobacco control policies on smoking cessation in high and low educated groups in 18 European countries. *Tobacco Control*, *17*: 248–255. Published online May 15, 2008.

Hong Kong — Kwok MK et al. (2008, August). Early life secondhand smoke exposure and serious infectious morbidity during the first eight years: Evidence from Hong Kong's "Children of 1997" birth cohort. *Tobacco Control*, *17*(4): 263–270. http://tobaccocontrol. bmj.com/cgi/content/abstract/ tc.2007 .023887v1. Accessed October 4, 2008.

Indonesia — Semba RD et al. (2008). Paternal smoking and increased risk of infant and under-5 child mortality in Indonesia. *American Journal of Public Health*. Published online February 28, 2008.

Italy — Valente P et al. (2007). Exposure to fine and ultrafine particles from secondhand smoke in public places before and after the smoking ban, Italy 2005. *Tobacco Control*, *16*(5): 312–317.

Latin America, Asia, and Africa — Bloch M et al. (2008). Tobacco use and secondhand smoke exposure during pregnancy: An investigative survey of women in 9 developing nations. *American Journal of Public Health*. Published online February 28, 2008.

Russia — Perlman F, Bobak M, Gilmore A, McKee M. (2007). Trends in the prevalence of smoking in Russia during the transition to a market economy. *Tobacco Control; 16*: 299–305.

United States — Thomas S et al. (2008). Population tobacco control interventions and their effects on social inequalities in smoking: Systematic review. *Tobacco Control*. Published online May 19, 2008.

How Much Research?
US National Library of Medicine, PubMed database. (N.d.). http://www.ncbi.nlm.nih.gov/ pubmed. Accessed July 14, 2008.

Comparative Research
Centers for Disease Control and Prevention. (2006). Tobacco related mortality. http://www .cdc.gov/tobacco/data_statistics/ fact_sheets/health_effects/ tobacco_related_mortality.htm. Accessed August 20, 2008.

Centers for Disease Control and Prevention. (2008a). Deaths: Preliminary data for 2006. *National Vital Statistics Report*, *56*(16): 17–20. http://www .cdc.gov/nchs/ pressroom/08newsreleases/ mortality2006.htm. Accessed October 4, 2008.

Centers for Disease Control and Prevention. (2008b). National

Center for Health Statistics: Stroke/cerebrovascular disease. http://www.cdc.gov/nchs/ fastats/stroke.htm. Accessed August 20, 2008.

Flegal KM et al. (2005). Excess deaths associated with underweight, overweight, and obesity. *Journal of the American Medical Association*, *293*(15): 1861–1867.

U.S. National Institutes of Health. (2008, February 5). Estimates of funding for various diseases, conditions, research areas, actual expenditures for 2007. http://www.nih.gov/ news/fundingresearchareas.htm. Accessed October 4, 2008.

CHAPTER 21: CAPACITY BUILDING
Quote
Confucius. (N.d.). *The analects attributed to Confucius [Kongfuzi], 551–479 BCE by Lao-Tse [Lao Zi]*. Translated by James Legge. UCLA Center for East Asian Studies. East Asian Studies Documents. http://www .international.ucla.edu/eas/ documents/lunyuCh2.htm. Accessed December 15, 2008.

Text
Damast A. (2008, July 24). Bloomberg, Gates team up to fight smoking. *Business Week*. http://www.businessweek.com/ bwdaily/dnflash/content/ jul2008/db20080723_845410.htm. Accessed September 2, 2008.

Gates, Bloomberg launch $375M anti-smoking campaign. (2008, July 23). *USA Today*. http://www.usatoday.com/ news/health/2008-07-23-smoking_N.htm. Accessed September 2, 2008.

Gates and Bloomberg unite in global fight against tobacco. (2008, July 24). *Medical News Today*. http://www .medicalnewstoday.com/ articles/116039.php. Accessed September 2, 2008.

Map
World Health Organization. (2008). *Report on the global tobacco epidemic, 2008: The MPOWER package*. Geneva: WHO.

Symbols
Thailand — Vateesatokit P. (2008, August 27). Personal communication.

United States — Tobacco Free Kids. (2005). A broken promise to our children. The 1998 state tobacco settlement seven years later. http://www .tobaccofreekids.org/reports/ settlements/2006/fullreport. pdf. Accessed August 27, 2008.

SOURCES

All Other Countries — WHO MPOWER Report. (2008).

Low-Income Countries Spend Thailand — Vateesatokit. (2008).

United States — Tobacco Free Kids. (2005).

All Other Countries — WHO MPOWER Report. (2008).

**CHAPTER 22:
WHO FRAMEWORK
Convention on Tobacco Control
Quote**
Cicero. (N.d.) *De Legibus* 3.3.8. The Latin Library. http://www .thelatinlibrary.com/cicero/ leg3.shtml. Accessed September 3, 2008.

Text
Guindon E, Boisclair D. (2003). Past, current and future trends in tobacco use. HNP discussion paper: Economics of tobacco control paper no. 6, Tobacco Free Initiative. Geneva: World Health Organization. http:// www1.worldbank.org/tobacco/ pdf/Guindon-Past,% 20current-%20whole.pdf. Accessed June 26, 2008.

Map
World Health Organization. (2008). Full list of signatories and parties to the WHO Framework Convention on Tobacco Control. http://www .who.int/fctc/signatories_ parties/en/index.html. Accessed January 22, 2009.

Anticipated Tobacco Industry Responses to the FCTC
American Cancer Society/ International Union for Cancer Control. (2006). The advocate's guide to legislative strategies. Tobacco Control Strategy Planning Guide #3. http://www .strategyguides.globalink.org/ pdfs/Legislative_Strategies.pdf. Accessed October 9, 2008.

Framework Convention Alliance. (2007). COP-2 Briefing paper: Implementing Article 5.3 – Protection of Tobacco Control Measures from Interference by the Tobacco Industry. http:// www.fctc.org/index.php? option=com_content&view =article&id=172:cop-2- briefing-paper-implementing- article-53-protection-of- tobacco-control-measures- from-interference-by-the- tobacco-industry-&catid=138: industry-interference&Itemid =162. Accessed October 9, 2008.

**File Folder
We Need to Move Away**
British American Tobacco. (2003, May 21). Response to adoption of WHO tobacco treaty. http://www.bat.com/ group/sites/uk__3mnfen.nsf/ vwPagesWebLive/DO726KYJ/ $FILE/medMD726LGS.pdf? openelement. Accessed September 3, 2008.

**CHAPTER 23:
SMOKE-FREE AREAS
Quote**
World Bank. (2002). Smokefree workplaces at a glance. www1 .worldbank.org/tobacco/AAG% 20SmokeFree%20Workplaces .pdf. Accessed October 5, 2008.

Text
Americans for Nonsmokers' Rights. (2005, August). Ventilation and air filtration: What air filtration companies and the tobacco industry are saying. http://www.no-smoke.org/ document.php?id=267. Accessed January 2009.

Americans for Nonsmokers' Rights. (2006, August). Patron surveys and consumer behavior. http://www.no-smoke.org/pdf/ patronsurveys.pdf. Accessed January 2009.

Quinet M, Orban M, Philippet C, Riffon A, Andrien M. (2003). Nonsmokers protection in restaurants and bars in Europe: A survey in five European countries. European Network for Smoking Prevention, Europe Against Cancer. http://www .fares.be/tabagisme/news/ surveyHorecaFinalReport.pdf. Accessed June 2005.

Raaijmakers T, van den Borne I. (2001). Cost-benefits of workplace smoking policies. In Fleitman S (ed.). Smokefree workplaces: Improving the health and well-being of people at work. European Status Report, European Network for Smoking Prevention. http:// www.ensp.org/reports.cfm. Accessed July 2005. Geneva: WHO.

Map
Global Smokefree Partnership, Global Voices Report, 2008. www .globalsmokefreepartnership.org.

World Health Organization. (2008). *WHO report on the global tobacco epidemic, 2008: The MPOWER package*, 25–28.

Symbol
WHO MPOWER Report. (2008), 25–28.

Smoking Ban in Restaurants, 2007
WHO MPOWER Report. (2008), 25–28.

No Loss of Restaurant and Bar Sales
California Board of Equalization. (1997–2004).

http://www.boe.ca.gov/news/ t11q97f.htm, http://www.boe .ca.gov/news/t11q98f.htm, http://www.boe.ca.gov/news/ t1q99f.htm, http://www.boe .ca.gov/news/t11q00f.htm, http://www.boe.ca.gov/news/ pdf/T11q01.pdf, http://www .boe.ca.gov/news/pdf/10t11q02 .pdf, http://www.boe.ca.gov/ news/pdf/t1_1Q03.pdf, http:// www.boe.ca.gov/news/pdf/ t1_1q04.pdf. Accessed July 2005.

Repace J. (2000, June). Can ventilation control second-hand smoke in the hospitality industry? Figure 3:34. Citing California Department of Health, California Board of Equalization. Before and after smoke-free laws first quarter taxable sales figures for restaurants and bars, state of California 1992–1999. http://www.repace.com. Accessed October 5, 2008.

Reduction in Nicotine Levels (median serum cotinine levels)
Third National Report on Human Exposure to Environmental Chemicals, 2005. Median Serum Cotinine Levels in Nonsmokers, by Age Group—National Health and Nutrition Examination Survey (NHANES), United States, 1988–1991 through 2001–2002. http://www.cdc .gov/exposurereport/pdf/ factsheet_general.pdf.

File Folder
Hieronimus J. (1992, October 22). Memorandum: Impact of workplace restrictions on consumption and incidence, Philip Morris, USA. Bates No.: 2023914280/4284. http://www .pmdocs.com/getallimg.asp?if= avpidx&DOCID=2023914280/ 4284. Accessed July 2005.

**Wows
China** — Ministry of Health, People's Republic of China. (2007, May). China Tobacco Control Report. Beijing. Cited in WHO MPOWER Report. (2008), 26.

Ireland — Mulcahy M et al. (2005). Secondhand smoke exposure and risk following the Irish smoking ban: An assessment of salivary cotinine concentrations in hotel workers and air nicotine levels in bars. *Tobacco Control*, 14(6): 384–388.

United States, 2007 — Stark MJ et al. (2007). The impact of clean indoor air exemptions and preemption policies on the prevalence of a tobacco-specific lung carcinogen among nonsmoking bar and restaurant workers. *American Journal of Public Health*, 97(8): 1457–1463.

**CHAPTER 24:
MARKETING BANS
Quote**
Saffer H. (2000). Tobacco advertising and promotion. In Jha P, Chaloupka FJ (eds.), *Tobacco control in developing countries*. Oxford: Oxford University Press.

Text
Assunta M, Chapman S. (2004a). The tobacco industry's accounts of refining indirect tobacco advertising in Malaysia. *Tobacco Control*, 13(Suppl 2): ii63–ii70.

Assunta M, Chapman S. (2004b). The world's most hostile environment: How the tobacco industry circumvented Singapore's advertising ban. *Tobacco Control*, 13(Suppl 2): ii51–ii57.

Carter SM. (2003). New frontier, new power: The retail environment in Australia's dark market. *Tobacco Control*, 12(Suppl 3): iii95–iii101.

Saffer H, Chaloupka F. (2000). The effect of tobacco advertising bans on tobacco consumption. *Journal of Health Economics*, 19: 1117–1137.

Sargent JD, Beach ML, Dalton MA, et al. (2004). Effect of parental R-rated movie restriction on adolescent smoking initiation: A prospective study. *Pediatrics*, 114: 149–156.

Wakefield M, Letcher T. (2002). My pack is cuter than your pack. *Tobacco Control*, 11: 154–156.

Wakefield M, Morley C, Horan JK, Cummings KM. (2002). The cigarette pack as image: New evidence from tobacco industry documents. *Tobacco Control*, 11(Suppl 1): I73–I80.

World Bank. (1999). *Curbing the epidemic: Governments and the economics of tobacco control*. Washington, DC: World Bank.

Map
World Health Organization. (2008). *WHO report on the global tobacco epidemic, 2008: The MPOWER package*. Geneva: WHO.

Symbol
WHO MPOWER Report. (2008).

Point-of-Sale Advertising Bans
WHO MPOWER Report. (2008).

Decline in Brand Recognition
Fielding R, Chee YY, Choi KM, Chu TK, Kato K, Lam SK, Sin KL, Tang KT, Wong HM, Wong KM. (2004). Declines in tobacco brand recognition and ever-smoking rates among young children following restrictions on tobacco advertisements in

Hong Kong. *Journal of Public Health*, 26(1): 24–30. DOI: 10.1093/pubmed/fdh118.

**Wows
Advertising Bans**
Blecher E. (2008). The impact of advertising bans on consumption in developing countries. *Journal of Health Economics*, 27: 930–942.

Upon Ratification
WHO Framework Convention on Tobacco Control. (2006). Tobacco advertising, promotion and sponsorship. Article 13/2: 8.

Comprehensive Advertising Bans
Saffer and Chaloupka. (2000).

**CHAPTER 25:
PRODUCT LABELING
Quote**
Simpson, D. (2004). Uganda: Official's "shock" over warning size. *Tobacco Control*, 13: 324.

Text
Borland R, Fong GT, Yong HH, Cummings KM, Hammond D, King B, Siahpush M, McNeill A, Hastings G, O'Connor RJ, Elton-Marshall T, Zanna MP. (2008). What happened to smokers' beliefs about light cigarettes when "light/mild" brand descriptors were banned in the UK? Findings from the International Tobacco Control (ITC) four-country survey. *Tobacco Control*. Published online first: April 21, 2008. doi:10.1136/ tc.2007.023812

Cunningham R. (2007). Package warnings: Overview of international developments. Canadian Cancer Society. http://www .smoke-free.ca/warnings/ WarningsResearch/Release_ WarningLabels_20070320.pdf. Accessed October 5, 2008.

Freeman B, Chapman S, Rimmer M. (2008). The case for the plain packaging of tobacco products. *Addiction*, 103(4): 580–590. http://tobacco.health.usyd.edu .au/site/futuretc/pdfs/generic .pdf. Accessed January 2009.

World Health Organization. (2005). Framework convention on tobacco control. Geneva: WHO/Tobacco-Free Initiative. http://www.who.int/fctc/ en/index.html. Accessed October 5, 2008.

World Health Organization. (2008). *WHO report on the global tobacco epidemic, 2008: The MPOWER package*. Geneva: WHO, 35.

Map
Tobacco Labelling Resource Centre. Country Information. http://www.tobaccolabels.ca/ currentl

WHO MPOWER Report. (2008), Q13.

Symbol
WHO MPOWER Report. (2008), Q14i.

Physicians for a Smoke-Free Canada. (N.d.). Health warnings with pictures are a very effective way to reduce smoking. http://www.smoke-free.ca/warnings. Accessed May 2, 2008.

Tobacco Labelling Resource Centre. (N.d.). Romania. http://www.igloo.org/community.igloo?r0=community&r0_script=/scripts/folder/view.script&r0_pathinfo=%2F%7Bf0ce20c6-7a3c-409a-a5c9-15e2b251a129%7D%2Fcurrentl%2Fromania&r0_output=xml. Accessed August 2008.

Misleading Lights
Physicians for a Smoke-Free Canada. (2005). Canadian Tobacco Use Monitoring Survey (CTUMS): A comprehensive plan to end the "light" and "mild" deception. http://www.smoke-free.ca/pdf_1/Endingthedeception-2005.pdf. Accessed October 5, 2008.

Bans on Terms Such as "Low Tar," "Light," "Ultra-Light," or "Mild."
WHO MPOWER Report. (2008), Q11.

File Folder
Chapman S, Carter SM. (2003). "Avoid health warnings on all tobacco products for just as long as we can": A history of Australian tobacco industry efforts to avoid, delay and dilute health warnings on cigarettes. *Tobacco Control*, 12(Suppl 3): iii13–iii22.

Wows
Plain Packaging
Freeman, Chapman, and Rimmer. (2008).

Health Warnings on Tobacco Packages
WHO MPOWER Report. (2008), 35.

CHAPTER 26: PUBLIC HEALTH CAMPAIGNS
Quote
Saloojee, Y. (2007). Presentation, 38th World Conference on Lung Health. Cape Town, South Africa.

Text
Asbridge M. (2004). Public place restrictions on smoking in Canada: assessing the role of the state, media, science and public health advocacy. *Social Science and Medicine* 58(1): 13–24.

Christakis NA, Fowler JH. (2008). The collective dynamics of smoking in a large social network. *New England Journal of Medicine*, 358(21): 2249–2258.

Annual Themes of World No Tobacco Day:
May 31, 1988–2008
World Health Organization. (N.d.). Tobacco Free Initiative (TFI). World No Tobacco Day. http://www.who.int/tobacco/resources/publications/wntd/en/. Accessed October 12, 2008.

Youth Prevention Programs
World Health Organization. (2002). Seeing beneath the surface: The truth about the tobacco industry's youth smoking prevention programmes. Tobacco Free Initiative: WHO Western Pacific Region Pamphlet. http://www.wpro.who.int/NR/rdonlyres/11EAD35E-741D-4736-B32D-300E85C29425/0/Seeingbeneaththesurface.pdf. Accessed October 12, 2008.

File Folder
Tobacco Institute. (1991, January 29). Discussion Paper. Bates No. TIMN0164422/4424 (see also TIFL0526381/6383). http://www.tobaccoinstitute.com/PDF/TIMN0164422_4424.PDF. Accessed October 18, 2008.

Wows
No Sensible, Ethical Person
World Health Organization Western Pacific Regional Office, Tobacco Free Initiative. (2002).

A Hallmark of All
Tobacco Free Kids. (2005). A long history of empty promises. The cigarette companies' ineffective youth anti-smoking programs. www.tobaccofreekids.org/research/factsheets/pdf/0010.pdf. Accessed October 12, 2008.

In the First Six Months
Graphic anti-smoking campaigns work. (2007, June 4). *ABC News* citing S. Stillman (acting director, QUIT, Australia). http://www.abc.net.au/news/stories/2007/06/04/1941268.htm. Accessed November 25, 2008.

CHAPTER 27: QUITTING SMOKING
Quote
Squires, S. (2002, February 19). The butt stops here. *Washington Post.* http://www.oralcancerfoundation.org/tobacco/butt_stops_here.htm. Accessed October 20, 2008.

Text
Anderson CM, Zhu S-H. (2007). Tobacco quitlines: Looking back and looking ahead. *Tobacco Control*, 16(Supplement 1): i81–i86. http://tobaccocontrol.bmj.com/cgi/content/full/16/Suppl_1/i81. Accessed September 1, 2008.

Peto R, Lopez AD. (2001). The future worldwide health effects of current smoking patterns. Pages 154–161 in *Critical Issues in Global Health*, Koop EC, Pearson CE, Schwarz MR (eds.). New York: Jossey-Bass.

World Health Organization. (2008). *WHO report on the global tobacco epidemic, 2008: The MPOWER package.* Geneva: WHO.

Map
Australia: Stanton, Harley. (2009). Personal communication.

WHO MPOWER Report. (2008).

Symbols
WHO MPOWER Report. (2008).

Tobacco Deaths
Peto and Lopez. (2001).

Why People Quit Smoking
Taylor T, Lader D, Bryant A, Keyse L, Joloza MT. (2005). Smoking-related behaviour and attitudes, 2005. http://www.statistics.gov.uk/downloads/theme_health/Smoking2005.pdf. Accessed June 4, 2008.

File Folder
Floridians to sue tobacco companies. (2007, September 26). WAWS Fox 30 News (Jacksonville, FL, USA). http://www.tobacco.org/news/252875.html. Accessed September 1, 2008.

Wows
China
Yang GH, Ma JM, Liu N, Zhou LN. (2005). Smoking and passive smoking in Chinese, 2002. *Zhonghua Liu Xing Bing Xue Za Zhi (Chinese Journal of Epidemiology)*, 26(2): 77–83.

Japan
Hirayama T. (1995). Personal communication.

Japan Tobacco. (1960–2005). Annual reports.

Mochizuki-Kobayashi Y. (2008). Personal communication.

CHAPTER 28: TOBACCO PRICES AND TAXES
Quote
Tobacco Free Initiative (TFI). (2005). Article 6: Price and tax measures to reduce the demand for tobacco. World Health Organization Framework Convention on Tobacco Control (WHO FCTC). http://www.who.int/tobacco/framework/final_text/en/index5.html. Accessed March 2, 2008.

Text
Jha P, Chaloupka F (eds.). (2000). *Tobacco control in developing countries.* New York: Oxford University Press.

Ross H, Chaloupka F. (2006). Economic policies for tobacco control in developing countries. *Journal Salud Publica de Mexico* 48(3): 113–120.

World Bank. (1999). *Curbing the epidemic: Governments and the economics of tobacco control.* Washington DC: World Bank Group.

Map
Albania, Bosnia and Herzegovina, Croatia, Moldova, Republic of, Montenegro, Norway, Serbia, Switzerland, Uzbekistan — World Health Organization. (2007). *The European tobacco control report: 2007.* Copenhagen: World Health Organization. http://www.euro.who.int/document/e89842.pdf.

Angola, Bahrain, Cuba, Djibouti, Egypt, Iran, Islamic Republic of, Korea, Republic of, Kuwait, Liberia, Libyan Arab Jamahiriya, Myanmar, Qatar, Sri Lanka, Syrian Arab Republic, Yemen — World Health Organization. (2008). *WHO report on the global tobacco epidemic, 2008: The MPOWER package.* Geneva: WHO.

Argentina, Bolivia, Brazil, Chile, Colombia, Lao People's Democratic Republic, Nepal — WHO MPOWER Report. (2008); VAT calculated from ERC. (2007). *World cigarette survey 2007.* London: ERC Group Plc.

Armenia, Algeria, Botswana, Burundi, Benin, Burkina Faso, Cape Verde, Central African Republic, Chad, Comoros, Congo, DRT Congo, Costa Rica, Cote D'ivoire, Dominica, Ecuador, El Salvador, Equatorial Guinea, Eritrea, Ethiopia, Gabon, Guatemala, Guinea, Guyana, Honduras, Jamaica, Jordan, Kenya, Lebanon, Lesotho, Malawi, Mali, Mauritania, Mauritius, Mozambique, Morocco, Nicaragua, Niger, Nigeria, Panama, Paraguay, Peru, Rwanda, Sao Tome And Principe, Senegal, Seychelles, Sierra Leone, South Africa, Suriname, Swaziland, Tanzania, United Republic of, Trinidad and Tobago, Togo, Turkmenistan, Uganda, Uruguay, Venezuela, Zambia, Zimbabwe — WHO MPOWER Report. (2008); VAT calculated from Deloitte. (2008). Global Indirect Tax Rates. http://www.deloitte.com/dtt/article/0,1002,cid%253D5028,00.html. Accessed May 30, 2008.

Australia — WHO MPOWER Report. (2008); VAT calculated from Euromonitor International. (2006). *The World Market for Tobacco.* Euromonitor International Inc.

Austria, Belgium, Bulgaria, Cyprus, Czech Republic, Denmark, Estonia, Finland, France, Germany, Greece, Hungary, Ireland, Italy, Latvia, Lithuania, Luxembourg, Malta, Netherlands, Poland, Portugal, Romania, Slovakia, Slovenia, Spain, Sweden, United Kingdom — EU Taxation and Customs Union. http://ec.europa.eu/taxation_customs/index_en.htm. Accessed December 13, 2008.

Bangladesh, Maldives, Oman, Saudi Arabia, United Arab Emirates — Guindon GE & Boisclair D. *Tobacco Taxation dataset 1999–2005.* Prepared for the American Cancer Society, Aug 2005. Perucic AM. *Tobacco Tax Earmarking dataset.* Prepared for the American Cancer Society; Aug 2005.

Barbados, Belarus, Dominican Republic, Kyrgyzstan, Namibia — Becker L. (2007, February). Developing Country Health Financing: Reverse the Decline of Tobacco Taxes; *Health Financing Task Force: Policy Brief.* http://resultsfordevelopment.org/_docs/febpolicybriefweb.pdf. Accessed November 26, 2008.

Cambodia — Ministry of Economy and Finance. (2006). Taxes on domestic goods and services. http://www.ocm.gov.kh/c_tax2.htm. Accessed December 15, 2008.

Canada — Physicians for a smoke-free Canada. (2008). http://www.smoke-free.ca/factsheets/pdf/Tobacco%20Tax%20Rates.pdf. Accessed May 30, 2008.

China — Hu T, Mao Z, Shi J. (2007). Tobacco taxation and its potential economic impact in China. A paper prepared for the Bloomberg Global Initiative to Reduce Tobacco Use Project. Unpublished manuscript.

Georgia — USAID. (2004). http://georgia.usaid.gov/pdf/18.pdf. Accessed May 30, 2008.

Ghana — ERC. (2007). *World cigarette survey 2007.* London: ERC Group Plc.

India — WHO MPOWER Report. (2008); VAT calculated from Sharma S. (July 21, 2007). ITC's cigarette sales are "under pressure" from value-added tax. Bloomberg.com. http://www.bloomberg.com/apps/news?pid=newsarchive&sid=aNDJY3KKh9.8. Accessed May 30, 2008.

SOURCES

Indonesia, Malaysia, Philippines, Thailand, Vietnam — ACS calculation by Hana Ross. (2008).

Israel — WHO MPOWER Report. (2008); VAT calculated from Worldwide Tax. (2008). Israel Tax News 2008. http://www.worldwide-tax.com/israel/isr_econonews.asp. Accessed May 30, 2008.

Japan — Kato T. (2008). Japan Tobacco falls on higher cigarette tax proposal. http://tobacco.cleartheair.org.hk/2008/06/06/japan-tobacco-falls-on-higher-cigarette-tax-proposal/. Accessed December 5, 2008.

Kazakhstan — Khakimzhanov, S. (2007). Estimation and simulation of tobacco excise increase in Kazakhstan. Unpublished manuscript.

Macedonia, Former Yugoslav Republic of — WHO MPOWER Report. (2008); VAT calculated from United States Council for International Business. (2008). Duties and Value-Added Taxes. http://www.uscib.org/index.asp?documentID=1676. Accessed May 30, 2008.

Mexico — Jimenez-Ruiz, J., Saenz de Miera, B., Reynales-Shigematsu, L., Waters, H., Hernandez-Avila, M. *The Impact of Taxation on Tobacco Consumption in Mexico.* Tobacco Control, 2008. 17 (2): p. 105–110.

Mongolia — WHO MPOWER Report. (2008); VAT calculated from International Publishers Association. (2006). http://www.ipa-uie.org/statistics/vat%20march%2006.htm. Accessed May 30, 2008.

New Zealand, Madagascar, Singapore, Cameroon — WHO MPOWER Report. (2008); VAT calculated from ERC. (2006). *World cigarette survey 2006.* London: ERC Group Plc.

Pakistan — Economics of tobacco for the South Asia (SA) region. 2001. http://siteresources.worldbank.org/INTETC/Resources/375990-1089913200558/SouthAsia.pdf. Accessed December 5, 2008.

Russian Federation — Ross H, Shariff S, Gilmore A. (In press). *Economics of tobacco taxation in Russia.* Baltimore: Bloomberg Initiative to Reduce Tobacco Use.

Turkey — Meric AB, Mulier T. (2008, February 22). BAT bids $1.72 billion to win Turkey's Tekel auction (Update 4). *Bloomberg News.* http://www.gab-ibn.com/IMG/pdf/Tr8-_BAT_Bids_1.72_Billion_to_Win_ Turkey_s_Tekel_Auction.pdf. Accessed November 26, 2008.

Tunisia — World Bank: Country Profiles. (2000). http://www1.worldbank.org/tobacco/pdf/country%20briefs/Tunisia.pdf. Accessed December 13, 2008.

Ukraine — Ross H, Shariff S, Gilmore A. (In press). *Economics of tobacco taxation in Ukraine.* Baltimore: Bloomberg Initiative to Reduce Tobacco Use.

United States of America — Campaign for Tobacco-Free Kids. (2008). State cigarette excise tax rates & rankings. http://www.tobaccofreekids.org/research/factsheets/pdf/0097.pdf. Accessed December 5, 2008.

Symbols
Economist Intelligence Unit. (N.d.). Worldwide cost of living survey. http://eiu.enumerate.com/asp/wcol_WCOLHome.asp. Accessed March 3, 2008.

World Bank. (2008). World Development Indicators. Washington DC: World Bank.

Smoking Goes Down
Aloui O. (2003). Analysis of the economics of tobacco in Morocco. Economics of Tobacco Control Paper No. 7. HNP Discussion Paper 2003. http://www1.worldbank.org/tobacco/pdf/Aloui-Analysis%20of%20-%20whole.pdf. Accessed March 1, 2008.

Tax Revenues Go Up
Walbeek C. (2003). Tobacco excise taxation in South Africa. WHO Tobacco Control Papers 2003. http://repositories.cdlib.org/tc/whotcp/SAfrica2003/. Accessed March 2, 2008.

Walbeek C. (2008). Personal communication.

File Folder
Chaloupka F. (2002). The role of tax increases in reducing consumption. http://www.impacteen.org/generalarea_PDFs/APHA2002_fjctobaccotax.pdf. Accessed March 1, 2008.

Wow
Hu T, Mao Z. (2002). Effects of cigarette tax on cigarette consumption and the Chinese economy. *Tobacco Control, 11:* 105–108.

CHAPTER 29: LITIGATION
Quote
United States vs. Philip Morris. (2006). Final opinion. http://www.usdoj.gov/civil/cases/tobacco2/amended%20opinion.pdf. Accessed October 13, 2008.

Text
Blanke DD. (2008). Towards health with justice: Litigation and public inquiries as tools for tobacco control. World Health Organization. http://www.who.int/tobacco/media/en/final_jordan_report.pdf. Accessed July 10, 2008.

Philip Morris International. (2008). Tobacco lawsuits outside the United States. http://www.philipmorrisinternational.com/PMINTL/pages/eng/busenv/Int_litigation.asp. Accessed August 5, 2008.

United States vs. Philip Morris. (2006).

World Health Organization. (2003). Framework Convention on Tobacco Control, World Health Organization. Geneva: WHO.

Map
Altadis Annual Report 2006. http://www.altadis.com/en/shareholders/pdf/meeting2007/2006AR-En.pdf. Accessed on June 16, 2008.

Altria Group, Inc. 2007 Annual Report. http://www.altria.com/AnnualReport/ar2007/2007ar_01_0100.aspx. Accessed on June 16, 2008.

British American Tobacco Annual Report and Accounts 2007. http://www.bat.com/annualreport2007. Accessed on August 22, 2008.

Gallaher Group Plc Interim Report 2006. http://ir.gallaher-group.com/downloads/ir/publications/2006_interim.pdf. Accessed June 16, 2008.

Imperial Tobacco Group PLC Annual Report and Accounts 2007. http://www.imperial-tobacco.com/files/financial/reports/ar2007/files/pdfs/itgar07_fullreport.pdf. Accessed June 16, 2008.

Japan Tobacco Inc. Annual Report 2007. http://www.jti.co.jp/JTI_E/IR/07/annual2007/annual2007_E_all.pdf. Accessed June 16, 2008.

Tobacco Control Legal Consortium: New Zealand High Court Dismisses Pioneering Tobacco Liability Case: http://www.wmitchell.edu/tobaccolaw/resources/LegalUpdate0506.pdf

A Range of Lawsuits
Altria Group Inc. (2007).

Cases Pending
Altria Group Inc. (2007).

British American Tobacco. (2007).

Gallaher Group Plc. (2006).

Imperial Tobacco Group Plc. (2007).

Japan Tobacco Inc. (2007).

Cases Pending Against Philip Morris
Altria Group Inc. (2007).

File Folder
Japan Tobacco Inc. (2007).

CHAPTER 30: RELIGION
Quote
BrainyQuote: Buddha Quotes. (N.d.). http://www.brainyquote.com/quotes/authors/b/buddha.html. Accessed December 4, 2008.

Text
American Heart Association. (2008). American Indians/Alaska Natives and cardiovascular diseases. Statistical fact sheet: 2008 update. http://www.americanheart.org/downloadable/heart/1199481493031FS02AM08.pdf. Accessed August 6, 2008.

American Lung Association. (2007, June). Smoking and American Indians/Alaska Natives Fact Sheet. http://www.lungusa.org/site/c.dvLUK9O0E/b.35999/k.EBAD/Smoking_and_American_IndiansAlaska_Natives_Fact_Sheet.htm. Accessed August 6, 2008.

Australian Broadcasting Corporation. (2002, May 8). Buddhist monks meet to tackle the issue of smoking. http://www.tobacco.org/news/93056.html. Accessed October 20, 2008.

Centers for Disease Control and Prevention. (1998). 1998 Surgeon General's report: Tobacco use among U.S. racial/ethnic minority groups: American Indians and Alaska Natives and Tobacco. http://www.cdc.gov/tobacco/data_statistics/sgr/sgr_1998/sgr-min-nat.htm. Accessed August 6, 2008.

U.S. Department of Health and Human Services. (2008). Indian Health Service. Division of Epidemiology and Disease Prevention. http://www.ihs.gov/medicalprograms/epi/index.cfm?module=health_issues&option=tobacco&cat=sub_0. Accessed October 17, 2008.

Winter JC. (2000). *Tobacco use by Native North Americans: Sacred smoke and silent killer.* Oklahoma City: University of Oklahoma Press.

World Council of Churches. (2000). Tobacco: A global problem requires a global response! http://www.oikoumene.org/fileadmin/files/wcc-main/documents/p4/contact/con-168.pdf. Accessed July 30, 2008.

World Health Organization. (1999). Meeting report: Meeting on tobacco and religion. www.who.int/entity/tobacco/media/en/religioneng.pdf. Accessed October 20, 2008.

Map
Central Intelligence Agency. (2008, October 9). The World Factbook: Field listing — religions. https://www.cia.gov/library/publications/the-world-factbook/fields/2122.html. Accessed October 17, 2008.

Foreign and Commonwealth Office. (2007). About the FCO: Country profiles. http://www.fco.gov.uk/en/about-the-fco/country-profiles/. Accessed October 17, 2008.

NationMaster. (2008). Nations of the world. http://www.nationmaster.com/index.php. Accessed July 30, 2008.

Religions
Central Intelligence Agency. (2008, October 9). The world factbook: World. https://www.cia.gov/library/publications/the-world-factbook/geos/xx.html#People. Accessed August 4, 2008.

Bahá'i Faith
The Bahá'i Faith, Substance Abuse and Addiction Treatment. (N.d.). Bahá'i scriptures on alcohol, tobacco and other drugs. http://bahaisofplainview.tripod.com/Bahais_and_Addictive_Illness/id3.html. Accessed August 4, 2008.

Bahá'i World Faith. (N.d.). Tablet on purity. http://www.bcca.org/ref/books/bwf/0717tabletonpurity.html. Accessed August 5, 2008.

Buddhism
Introduction to Buddhism. (2008). http://www.buddhanet.net/e-learning/intro_bud.htm. Accessed July 22, 2008.

World Health Organization. (1999).

World Health Organization. (2002). International workshop on Buddhism and tobacco control, May 7–9, 2002. http://www.who.int/tobacco/national_capacity/religion/en. Accessed October 17, 2008.

Yel D, Hallen GK, Sinclair RG, Mom K, Srey CT. (2005). Biochemical validation of self-reported quit rates among Buddhist monks in Cambodia. *Tobacco Control, 14:* 359.

Christianity
World Council of Churches. (2000).

Church of Jesus Christ of Latter-Day Saints (Mormons)
The Church of Jesus Christ of Latter-Day Saints. (2008). Country profiles: USA-Utah. http://www.newsroom.lds.org/ldsnewsroom/eng/contact-us/usa-utah. Accessed August 4, 2008.

The Doctrine and Covenants of the Church of Jesus Christ of Latter-Day Saints, Section 89. (N.d.). http://scriptures.lds.org/dc/89. Accessed July 22, 2008.

Kaiser Family. (2008). State health facts: Utah. http://www.statehealthfacts.org/profileind.jsp?ind=80&cat=2&rgn=46. Accessed August 4, 2008.

Merrill RM, Lyon JL. (2005). Cancer incidence among Mormons and non-Mormons in Utah (United States), 1995–1999. *Preventive Medicine*, 40(5): 535–541.

Hinduism
World Health Organization. (1999).

Islam
Contemporary legal rulings in Shiëi law. (N.d.). Muëamalat (part 4) — Medical students. http://www.sistani.org/local.php?modules=nav&nid=2&bid=61&pid=3216&hl=smoking. Accessed July 22, 2008.

Khayat MH (ed.). (2000). *Islamic ruling on smoking*. Alexandria: World Health Organization, Regional Office of the Eastern Mediterranean.

World Health Organization. (1999).

World Health Organization Regional Office for the Eastern Mediterranean. (2006). Religion and tobacco: Together for tobacco free hajj. http://www.emro.who.int/TFI/TobaccofreeMecca_Medina.htm. Accessed August 5, 2008.

Judaism
Rabbinical Council of America. (2006, July 3). "RCA's Vaad Halacha bans use of tobacco products." http://www.rabbis.org/news/article.cfm?id=100808. Accessed August 5, 2008.

Siegel-Itzkovich J. (2008, July 7). Halachic ruling forbids smoking, calls for preventive health checkups. *Jerusalem Post*. http://www.jpost.com/servlet/Satellite?pagename=JPost/JPArticle/ShowFull&cid=1215530889024. Accessed August 5, 2008.

World Health Organization. (1999).

Roman Catholicism
Proceedings of the Papal Meetings. (2002). http://www.emro.who.int/TFI/vaticaneng.pdf. Accessed August 4, 2008.

World Health Organization. (1999).

Sikhism
Dhillon BS. (1998). Sikhism and smoking. http://www.sikhs.org/art9.htm. Accessed August 4, 2008.

Wows
Offering Cigarettes to Monks
Vateesatokit P. (2003). Tailoring tobacco control efforts to the country: The example of Thailand. Pages 154–178 in *Tobacco control policy: Strategies, successes, and setbacks*. J. de Beyer and L. V. Brigden (eds.). Washington, DC: World Bank.

Since the Damage Caused
Excerpts from the opinions of Muslim scholars concerning the Islamic ruling on smoking. (N.d.). World Health Organization: Tobacco and religion. http://www.emro.who.int/Publications/HealthEdReligion/Smoking/Excerpts.htm. Accessed October 17, 2008.

If Smoking Causes
Contemporary legal rulings in Shiëi law. (N.d.).

CHAPTER 31: THE FUTURE
Quote
World Health Organization. (2008a). *WHO report on the global tobacco epidemic, 2008: The MPOWER package*. Geneva: WHO. http://www.who.int/tobacco/mpower/mpower_report_full_2008.pdf. Accessed April 4, 2008.

Text
WHO MPOWER Report (2008a). Executive summary, 2.

Numbers of Smokers
Future Scenarios Plenary. (2000). Tobacco control 2015: Where, why and with what outcomes? 11th World Conference on Tobacco or Health. Chicago, Illinois, August 6–11, 2000.

Guindon E. (2002, June 3), WHO/EIP. Personal communication.

Mackay J. (1997). Lessons from the conference: The next 25 years. 10th World Conference on Tobacco or Health. Beijing, China, August 24–28, 1997.

Health, 2000–2010
World Health Organization. (2002). *The World Health Report 2002: Reducing risks, promoting healthy life*. Geneva: WHO, 65.

World Health Organization. (2008b). Tobacco-Free Initiative.

www.who.int/entity/tobacco/en/. Accessed February 9, 2008.

World Health Organization. (2008c). Fact sheet: 10 facts about tobacco and second-hand smoke. http://www.who.int/features/factfiles/tobacco/en/index.html. Accessed February 9, 2008.

Health, 2010–2020
Mathers CD, Loncar D. (2006, November). Projections of global mortality and burden of disease from 2002 to 2030. *PLoS Medicine* 3(11): e442.

World Health Organization. (2008b).

Health, 2020–2030
World Health Organization. (2008c).

Health, 2030–2040
World Health Organization. Tobacco Free Initiative. http://www.who.int/tobacco/en/ Accessed December 15, 2008.

World Health Organization. (2002). *The World Health Report 2002: Reducing risks, promoting healthy life*. Geneva: WHO, 65.

Health, 2040–2050
Lopez A. (2002, April 12). Personal communication, citing Peto R, Lopez A. (2001). The future worldwide health effects of current smoking patterns. Pages 154–161 in Koop EC, Pearson C, Schwarz P (eds.). *Global health in the 21st century*. New York: Jossey-Bass.

CHAPTER 32: THE HISTORY OF TOBACCO
Borio G. (N.d.). Tobacco timeline. http://www.tobacco.org/resources/history/Tobacco_History.html. Accessed December 15, 2008.

Cochran S. (1980). *Big business in China: Sino-foreign rivalry in the cigarette industry, 1890–1930*. Cambridge, MA: Harvard University Press.

Framingham Heart Study. (N.d.). A timeline of milestones. http://www.framingham.com/heart/timeline.htm. Accessed December 15, 2008.

Globalink. Tobaccopedia. (N.d.). http://tobaccopedia.org. Accessed July 16, 2005.

Kluger R. (1996). *Ashes to ashes: America's hundred-year war, the public health, and the unabashed triumph of Philip Morris*. New York: Alfred A Knopf.

Hong-Gwan S. (2005, August 1). Personal communication with chairman of Smoking Cessation Clinic, National Cancer Center, Republic of Korea.

Lyons AS, Petrucelli RJ. (1978). *Medicine: An illustrated history*. New York: Harry N. Abrams Inc., 508.

Moyer D. (1998). The tobacco almanac: A reference book of fact, figures, quotations about tobacco. (Self-published).

Routh HB, Bhowmik KR, Parish JL, Parish LC. (1998). Historical aspects of tobacco use and smoking. *Clinics in Dermatology* 16(5): 539–544.

James Walton (ed.). (2000). *The Faber book of smoking*. London: Faber.

Tobacco milestones: A brief history of tobacco. (1996). Adapted from a chronology by the National Clearinghouse on Tobacco and Health, Ottawa, Canada.

Tobacco Facts. (N.d.). Tobacco truth: From first drag to slavery: tobacco's beginnings. http://www.tobaccofacts.org/tob_truth/timeline1492.html. Accessed December 15, 2008.

PART SIX: WORLD TABLES
"No more hookah parlours in city." (July 5, 2008). *The Times of India*. Mumbai.

USEFUL CONTACTS

Online
Tobacco Atlas:
www.TobaccoAtlas.org

WHO Tobacco Free Initiative
WHO Headquarters
http://tobacco.who.int/

AFRO
http://www.afro.who.int/tfi/index.html

EMRO
http://www.emro.who.int/tfi/tfi.htm

EURO
http://www.euro.who.int/healthtopics/HT2
ndLvlPage?HTCode=tobacco
http://data.euro.who.int/tobacco/

PAHO
http://www.paho.org/english/ad/sde/ra/
tobdefault.htm

SEARO
http://www.searo.who.int/EN/Section1174/
Section2469.htm

WPRO
http://www.wpro.who.int/health_topics/
tobacco/

International Organizations

Action on Smoking and Health
http://www.newash.org.uk/

American Cancer Society
http://www.cancer.org/international

The Bloomberg Initiative to Reduce Tobacco Use
www.tobaccocontrolgrants.org/

British American Tobacco Document Collection
http://www.library.ucsf.edu/tobacco/batco/

Campaign for Tobacco-Free Kids
http://www.tobaccofreekids.org/
http://www.tobaccofreecenter.org/

Centers for Disease Control and Prevention (CDC)
http://www.cdc.gov/tobacco/global/

Corporate Accountability International
http://www.stopcorporateabuse.org/cms/
page1111.cfm

Doctors and Tobacco
http://www.doctorsandtobacco.org/
http://www.tobacco-control.org/

Framework Convention Alliance for Tobacco Control (FCA)
http://www.fctc.org/

FCTCnow!
http://www.fctcnow.org

FDI World Dental Federation
http://www.fdiworldental.org

Fogarty International Center
http://www.fic.nih.gov/index.htm

Global Dialogue for Effective Stop Smoking Campaigns
http://www.stopsmokingcampaigns
.org/index.php

GLOBALink: The International Tobacco Control Community
http://www.globalink.org/
http://gallery.globalink.org
http://petitions.globalink.org
http://news.globalink.org (English/
French/German/Spanish/Italian news
and information)

Global Partnerships for Tobacco Control
http://www.essentialaction.org/tobacco/

Global Smokefree Partnership
http://www.globalsmokefree.com/

Hamann's research site (Stephen Hamann)
http://hamann.globalink.org/

InterAmerican Heart Foundation - affiliates in Argentina, Jamaica, Mexico
www.interamericanheart.org

International Development Research Centre - Research for International Tobacco Control
www.idrc.ca/tobacco

International Network of Women Against Tobacco (INWAT)
http://www.inwat.org/

International Network Towards Smoke-Free Hospitals (INTSH)
http://intsh.globalink.org/

International Non Governmental Coalition Against Tobacco (INGCAT)
http://www.ingcat.org/

International Society for the Prevention of Tobacco Induced Diseases (PTID)
http://isptid.globalink.org/

International Tobacco Evidence Network (ITEN)
http://www.tobaccoevidence.net/

International Union Against Tuberculosis and Lung Disease (The Union)
http://www.tobaccofreeunion.org/

Johns Hopkins Bloomberg School of Public Health: Global Tobacco Control
http://www.globaltobaccocontrol.org/

Legacy Foundation, UCSF tobacco document site
http://legacy.library.ucsf.edu

London School of Hygiene and Tropical Medicine, University of London, Tobacco Control Research
http://www.lshtm.ac.uk/cgch/tobacco/

Pharmacists Against Tobacco
http://www.fip.org/projectsfip//
pharmacistsagainsttobacco/

Repace Associates Inc. Secondhand Smoke Consultants
http://www.repace.com/

Smokescreen Consulting
http://www.smokescreen.org

Smoke-Free Movies
http://www.smokefreemovies.ucsf.edu/
http://www.smoke-free.ca/movies/index
.htm

Society for Research on Nicotine and Tobacco (SRNT)
http://www.srnt.org/

Stanford School of Medicine—Images from the Tobacco Industry Campaign to Hide the Hazards of Smoking
http://lane.stanford.edu/tobacco/index
.html

Tobacco Academy
http://www.tobaccoacademy.org/

Tobacco Archives
http://www.tobaccoarchives.com/

Tobacco Control Archives—UCSF
http://www.library.ucsf.edu/tobacco/

Tobacco Control Journal
http://www.tobaccocontrol.com

Tobacco Control Supersite (Simon Chapman) - University of Sydney
http://www.health.usyd.edu.au/tobacco/

Tobacco Documents Online
http://www.tobaccodocuments.org

Tobacco.org—Tobacco news and information
http://www.tobacco.org

Tobacco Products Liability Project (TPLP)
http://tobacco.neu.edu/

Treatobacco Resources for Treatment of Tobacco Dependence, Society for Research on Nicotine and Tobacco/ International Union Against Cancer
http://www.treatobacco.net/

University of California, San Francisco (UCSF): Tobacco Control
http://tobacco.ucsf.edu/

World Conferences on Tobacco OR Health (GLOBALink resource)
http://www.wctoh.org

World Lung Foundation
http://www.worldlungfoundation.org

Regional Organizations

European Medical Association on Smoking and Health (EMASH)
http://emash.globalink.org/

European Network of Quitlines
http://www.enqonline.org/

European Network for Smoke-free Hospitals (ENSH)
http://ensh.aphp.fr/

European Network for Smoking Prevention (ENSP)
http://www.ensp.org

European Network of Young People and Tobacco
http://www.ktl.fi/enypat/

European Respiratory Society
http://dev.ersnet.org/

Southeast Asia Tobacco Control Alliance
http://www.seatca.org/

Syrian Center For Tobacco Studies
http://www.scts-sy.org/en/home.php

These Web addresses were active in mid-2008. There are many other national and subnational organizations, wholly or partly working on tobacco control issues, too numerous to include here. These can be located through INGCAT (the International Non Governmental Coalition Against Tobacco) or GLOBALink. If any would like to be included in future editions, or on a Web site, please contact the authors.

INDEX

INDEX